SAGE was founded in 1965 by Sara Miller McCune to support the dissemination of usable knowledge by publishing innovative and high-quality research and teaching content. Today, we publish over 900 journals, including those of more than 400 learned societies, more than 800 new books per year, and a growing range of library products including archives, data, case studies, reports, and video. SAGE remains majority-owned by our founder, and after Sara's lifetime will become owned by a charitable trust that secures our continued independence.

Los Angeles | London | New Delhi | Singapore | Washington DC | Melbourne

CULTURAL PSYCHOLOGY
OF HEALTH IN INDIA

CULTURAL PSYCHOLOGY OF HEALTH IN INDIA

Well-being, Medicine and Traditional Health Care

AJIT K DALAL

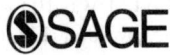

Los Angeles | London | New Delhi
Singapore | Washington DC | Melbourne

First published in 2016 by

SAGE Publications India Pvt Ltd
B1/I-1 Mohan Cooperative Industrial Area
Mathura Road, New Delhi 110 044, India
www.sagepub.in

SAGE Publications Inc
2455 Teller Road
Thousand Oaks, California 91320, USA

SAGE Publications Ltd
1 Oliver's Yard, 55 City Road
London EC1Y 1SP, United Kingdom

SAGE Publications Asia-Pacific Pte Ltd
3 Church Street
#10-04 Samsung Hub
Singapore 049483

Published by Vivek Mehra for SAGE Publications India Pvt Ltd, typeset in 10.5/12.5 pts Adobe Garamond Pro by Diligent Typesetter India Pvt Ltd, Delhi and printed at Saurabh Printers Pvt Ltd, Greater Noida.

Library of Congress Cataloging-in-Publication Data

Name: Dalal, Ajit K, author.
Title: Cultural psychology of health in India: well-being, medicine and traditional health care / Ajit K Dalal.
Description: New Delhi, India; Thousand Oaks, California: SAGE Publications India Pvt Ltd, 2016. | Includes bibliographical references and index.
Identifiers: LCCN 2016013836 | ISBN 9789351509806 (hardback: alk. paper) | ISBN 9789351509790 (epub) | ISBN 9789351509813 (ebook)
Subjects: | MESH: Psychology, Medical | Ethnopsychology | Medicine, Traditional | India—ethnology
Classification: LCC RC451.I6 | NLM WB 104 | DDC 616.8900954—dc23 LC record available at https://lccn.loc.gov/2016013836

ISBN: 978-93-515-0980-6 (HB)

SAGE Team: Shambhu Sahu, Alekha Chandra Jena and Ritu Chopra

To my teachers
Professor Ramadhar Singh,
Professor Janak Pandey and
Late Professor Mohan Chandra Joshi,
who have shaped my academic career.

Thank you for choosing a SAGE product!
If you have any comment, observation or feedback,
I would like to personally hear from you.
Please write to me at **contactceo@sagepub.in**

Vivek Mehra, Managing Director and CEO,
SAGE Publications India Pvt Ltd, New Delhi

Bulk Sales

SAGE India offers special discounts
for purchase of books in bulk.
We also make available special imprints
and excerpts from our books on demand.

For orders and enquiries, write to us at

Marketing Department
SAGE Publications India Pvt Ltd
B1/I-1, Mohan Cooperative Industrial Area
Mathura Road, Post Bag 7
New Delhi 110044, India

E-mail us at **marketing@sagepub.in**

Get to know more about SAGE

Be invited to SAGE events, get on our mailing list.
Write today to **marketing@sagepub.in**

This book is also available as an e-book.

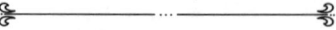

Contents

List of Abbreviations

ADD	Action for Disability and Development
AM	Alternative Medicine
ASHAs	Accredited Social Health Activists
AYUSH	Ayurveda, Yoga and Naturopathy, Unāni, Siddha and Homoeopathy
CBR	Community-based Rehabilitation
CHC	Community Health Centre
CHD	Coronary Heart Disease
CHW	Community Health Worker
CII	Confederation of Indian Industry
DABB	Disability Attitude Belief Behaviour
FDI	Foreign Direct Investment
ICF	International Classification of Functioning Disability and Health
ICU	Intensive Care Unit
IMR	Infant Mortality Rate
ILO	International Labour Organization
ISM	Indian Systems of Medicine
ISM&H	Indian Systems of Medicine and Homoeopathy
NREGS	National Rural Employment Guarantee Scheme
NCEUS	National Commission for Enterprises in the Unorganized Sector
NCPEDP	National Centre for Promotion of Employment for Disabled People
NGO	Non-governmental Organizations
NPC	National Planning Committee

NRHM	National Rural Health Mission
NSS	National Sample Survey of India
PHC	Primary Health Centre
RAHIS	Rajiv Aarogyasri Health Insurance Scheme
RCI	Rehabilitation Council of India
SHGs	Self-help Groups
SNS	Sympathetic Nervous System

Preface

Cultural Psychology of Health in India deals with the rapidly growing field of research on health and well-being from a cultural–psychological perspective. It examines the health care systems of India, which have evolved in different historical contexts, building on the then prevailing values, traditions and ethos of the society. Specifically, the book highlights and compares two diverse streams of health care—modern medicine and Indian systems—for their complementary role in providing affordable services in India. The six chapters included in this volume have been written at different points of time but have been updated and synchronized with the main theme of this volume.

Culture is a dynamic system of meanings and symbols which shapes every domain of our life. It provides a world view that gives meaning to personal and collective experiences and helps us in locating ourselves in the world we live. It affects our perceptions of health, illness and well-being, beliefs about causes of disease, approaches to health promotion, experience and expression of illness, help-seeking and the types of treatment sought. In the Western societies, for example, diseases are believed to be caused by microorganisms or bodily impairment and treatment is sought accordingly. In India, supernatural phenomena are also believed to cause diseases and divine intervention is sought. Here, multiple health care systems have flourished in the long history of three millennia; and pragmatic Indian ethos has carved space for indigenous and alien systems. The traditional Indian society has focused on the larger domain of suffering–healing while dealing with the physical and mental health issues. Modern medicine, which is presently the most dominant system of health care in India, has largely confined itself to physical health problems and their treatment. Traditional systems have an important role in providing holistic health care. Eventually, modern medicine may become part of the multi-coloured mosaic of health care systems in India.

The six chapters of this volume cover different sub-themes. The first chapter draws on the broad domain of cultural psychology of health. It provides a comparative view of modern and traditional Indian systems, examining health from both Western and Indian perspectives. The second chapter traces the history of Ayurveda and folk practices as well as their competitive but peaceful existence as complementary systems. The characteristic features of the indigenous systems have been highlighted. The third chapter discusses folk-healing systems in detail, describing the kind of important services the folk/faith healers are rendering across the country. Their healing practices are flexible and have undergone change with time and place but work within some broad guiding principles. The fourth chapter examines the possibilities of modern medicine and traditional systems operating as complementary systems, rather in contravention. The fifth chapter is about participatory rehabilitation of the poor with disability. The chapter deals with physical and psychosocial barriers in the mainstreaming of the disabled people. It also elaborates on the nexus between poverty and disability and suggests a participatory developmental model to improve their quality of life. The last chapter pertains to methodological issues in the research on cultural psychology of health. Broad methodological challenges of doing research in this emerging field have also been discussed. The chapter builds a case for yoga as an alternative research methodology for studying one's own physical, mental and spiritual health.

Overall, the volume has attempted to combine theoretical and practical issues with an objective to find viable solutions to India's massive health care challenge. There are no easy solutions. It is hoped that the coverage and critical analysis of the subject matter in various chapters will inspire readers to carry this debate further towards a logical end. India's public health care system is rapidly down-sliding and we need to think of innovative ways to rejuvenate it. This work should provide insights into how psychologists and other social scientists may play an active role, along with medical and traditional practitioners, in improving India's health.

This volume is a culmination of the work I started almost three decades back with a personal experience of long-term hospitalization. My earlier book *Health Beliefs and Coping with Chronic Diseases* (2015) lays groundwork on which this volume builds its thesis. Taken together, these two publications should present a comprehensive picture of how psychological factors are important considerations in providing complete health care to people. There is much to learn from traditional systems in this regard, as these two volumes clearly highlight.

The present volume should be a critical reading for students and researchers in the area of health psychology as well as for health practitioners, activists and writers. The volume is written in a manner that a layman can easily comprehend the first five chapters. The last chapter is intended more for researchers in the field of health and well-being.

I thank all those who have commented on the earlier versions of these chapters. I had presented some of these chapters in conferences and seminars, and was hugely benefitted from the constructive comments of the audience. I am equally grateful to my colleagues and friends, without naming anyone in particular, with whom I had extensive discussion on initial drafts of these chapters. They all have contributed in preparing the final version of this manuscript.

Udaipur   **Ajit K Dalal**

1

Cultural Psychology of Health and Well-being

In its quest to be a universal science, research in psychology has almost ignored culture as a legitimate field of investigation for a long time. The focus was on identifying universal attributes of human behaviour and developing theories and explanations applicable across cultures. In fact, the mainstream psychology, particularly the Western psychology, found culture as problematic in its pursuit to be scientific and empirical. For a long time, culture has been treated as some objectively bounded condition, like geographical region, and comparisons have been made between people of different nationalities. The research in this area expanded by taking an extended definition of culture in which attributes such as religion, caste, language and ethnicity were included. Culture becomes the basis to differentiate human groups and also the basis to explain and predict behaviour (Kazarian & Evans, 2001). A more relativistic position, taken in later years, focused on the meaning and functions of cultural symbols as embodied in social transactions and individual behaviour. It led to the development of culturally grounded theories in various fields of psychology. Contemporary research in psychology holds that individual and culture are bound in a close symbiotic relation. In the socialization process, cultural meanings of objects and concepts are internalized by its members, as at the same time, new meanings and patterns of behaviour emerge in social interaction (Miller, 1997; Valsiner, 2007). People can be classified as belonging to different cultures, and at the same time, culture is viewed as a system that organizes psychological world of individuals. Cultural psychology thus encompasses beliefs, attitudes, knowledge, traditions, symbols, customs, ethics, morals, social institutions and shared history which shape and are shaped by collective behaviour of people in a particular society.

Quite often the terms ethnic, folk, traditional, indigenous and cultural psychology are used interchangeably. Psychological research and writings in these areas overlap in conceptualization and coverage of the subject matter. Much is written on the cultural aspects of human behaviour in the present times. German scholar, Wilhelm Wundt, who is credited with the first psychology laboratory at Leipzig, Germany, in 1879, was also a pioneer in the field of cultural psychology. It is little known that he wrote in the period 1910–1920, a ten-volume long treatise on the *Völkerpsychologie* (cultural psychology). He compiled and integrated social theories, customs, traditions, beliefs and practices of the Western world and scientifically analyzed them. He examined the meaning of cultural artefacts and language, and endeavoured to understand higher-order mental processes, while leaving the basic processes to experimental psychological inquiries (Shiraev, 2010). Unfortunately, his important contribution was completely ignored by his contemporary and later psychologists in their pursuit to promote experimental tradition. Culture as an important consideration in psychological research was resurrected only in last decades of the past century.

Following Descartenian logic of mind–body dichotomy, historically a differentiation was made between physical and mental health, consequently leaving physical health in the hands of medical professionals. Clinical psychology developed as a new branch of psychology to diagnose mental pathologies and psychotherapies. Freudian psychoanalysis contributed significantly in the development of this field. At the same time, it was acknowledged by many health practitioners that specific organic illnesses are the result of mental conflicts and personality disorders. Dunbar (1943), for example, argued that conflicts produce anxiety which becomes unconscious and causes ulcer. His and other work in this area gave rise to a new branch of psychosomatic medicine. This development was reassertion of the age-old belief that mind and body closely interact, and that bodily diseases are caused by the mental state. Research accumulated over the years to establish that psychological variables play a vital role both in causing and recovering from illness and also in maintaining good health. This led to the emergence of a new discipline of health psychology (Taylor, 2006). Presently, health psychology is the most rapidly growing branch of psychology all over the world.

It is only in the last two decades that health psychologists started getting engaged in cultural imperatives of health. Anthropological work has examined health and healing practices of different regions of the world and provided evidences of their efficacy in dealing with many mental and physical health problems (Kleinman, 1987). This line of work got many health psychologists interested in more thoroughly examining the cultural aspects of health. Another compelling factor was that with heavy influx of immigrants, Western societies were becoming multicultural (Mather, 2009). To deal with health problems of immigrants, it was realized that knowledge about their native culture was necessary. Many indigenous health care practices were also brought along by the immigrants, which now constitute a part of the alternative medicinal system. Today, with high population mobility across the globe, all major countries of the world are turning multicultural. Alternative health care practices are now accepted and practised by a wide cross section of the population. The third factor behind the emergence of cultural psychology of health was defining health in terms of 'well-being'. This broad definition covers all the aspects of health, including positive and growth-related ones which are often contingent on their cultural beliefs, values and practices. In this backdrop, the cultural psychology of health is that branch of psychology which deals with culturally determined health behaviour and well-being.

The notion that psychological state influences the health status of a person has a long history in the Indian healing system. The ancient Vedic texts proposed an essential unity of the mind and the body and delineated theories and practices to deal with a large number of health-related problems. The Atharvaveda and the Yajurveda provide ample descriptions of a variety of physical and mental disorders and the course of treatment (Mondal, 1996). In Ayurveda (the science of life), health and well-being are understood in a holistic manner in which physical, mental, social and spiritual factors are closely intertwined. Medical practitioners from other cultures came to India at different points of time in history and found it a congenial place to practise their system of healing. In present times, the plural health care system of India offers a wide variety of treatment options to patients.

This essay discusses the development of the cultural psychology of health as an independent academic discipline. It brings out the salient features of biomedical and Ayurvedic system of medicine in light of a comprehensive holistic model of health and well-being. The essay examines how personality, affective and cultural factors shape the health status of a person. It explores the possibility of integrating cultural and psychological factors in the proposed psychomedical model of health care.

Health Psychology as a Forerunner

In the last 3–4 decades, the field of health psychology has grown rapidly with the realization that mind and body are closely intertwined and that human health needs to be viewed from the psychosocial perspective as well. Staying healthy is dependent, not only on good physic but also on health habits, life orientation, attitudes and beliefs, social support and emotional state. This stance led to the development of a biopsychosocial model of health care, which was later articulated and elaborated by Engel (1977). In this alternative model, apart from physical condition of the person, Engel included patient's personal experiences and social or cultural context into a more comprehensive framework for understanding disease, illness and health. Engel's model holds that psychosocial factors are crucial in not only restoring good health but also preventing diseases and promoting good health.

Research in the field of health psychology proliferated in which endeavour was to identify psychosocial causes of diseases from which people suffer. Personality, motivational, affective and behavioural factors were identified leading to a host of physical diseases. For example, prolonged psychological stress was found to be responsible for hypertension, peptic ulcer and many other diseases. Psychosocial factors were also found important in the recovery from the physical ailments. Research in the areas of patient compliance, doctor–patient communication, hospital environment and nursing care has yielded rich data to improve health services and to create better treatment conditions. Research in these areas carved out a role for psychologists to improve health status of the masses. They can also play a role in augmenting public health care programmes and contribute in improving the quality of life and well-being in the society.

Clinical psychology as a sister discipline of health psychology has failed to fulfil this role. Being in existence for more than 100 years, clinical psychology confined itself to the study of classification of mental illnesses, aetiology, diagnosis and treatment of the afflicted patients. Conforming to mind–body dualism, clinical psychologists only focused on mental health problems. Working in a clinical setting, their role remained subsidiary to those of the psychiatrists. Confined to mental health-related issues, clinical psychologists were largely ill-equipped to understand the psychological aspects of physical health problems. Health psychology was officially recognized as a separate branch of psychology by the American Psychological Association and a separate Division 38 was created in 1978. Health psychology grew in strength with the conviction that patients are not merely passive recipients of a certain treatment regimen, but should be considered as equal partners to achieve the common goal of (better) health (Adler, 2009).

Health psychology primarily remained part of the mainstream psychology and only marginally paid attention to its cultural moorings. Research publications in health psychology journals have rarely focused on cultural issues. Even though the salience of culture in human behaviour in general, and health in particular, has been acknowledged, the scientific research on health primarily focused on individual level variables. In the prevalent biomedical model of health, culture was not seen as a critical consideration in understanding and changing health behaviour. The role of culture was ignored in developing effective strategies for the treatment and prevention of illnesses, for health promotion, for improving the quality of life, for the training of health professionals and for formulating health care policy in plural societies. Taking the cultural perspective of health holds the promise of understanding health, illness and well-being in terms of traditions, beliefs and practices of a community. It would help in moving out of the individual-centred approach to health, situating health in the much larger domain and involving all stakeholders.

Emergence of Cultural Psychology of Health

The emerging discipline of cultural psychology of health and well-being has grown on the meaningful integration of the knowledge from the fields of health psychology and cultural psychology. These resources are required to familiarize researchers, practitioners and students in the field of health with the role of culture in the science, practice and training of health care. The availability of conceptual frameworks and theoretical frameworks is still inadequate to interface between health behaviour and culture. The integration of the cultural perspective into health psychology research is imperative for examining alternative models of health care and for developing holistic health practices. Health research in psychology is still in a nascent state of development, and we still have a long way to go to alleviated human suffering and promote psychological well-being.

In the recent past, culture in health and well-being has been examined from three perspectives: cross-cultural, cultural and indigenous. In cross-cultural perspective, culture is conceptualized as an independent variable where culture is treated as a variable to compare two or more cultural groups to identify similarities and differences. Conceptual and operational equivalence of health-related variables in the study is first established for cross-cultural comparison (Berry, 2000). Cultural psychology, which emerged later, considers culture and behaviour as inseparable and behaviour is seen only in relation to a culture (Kitayama & Cohen, 2007; Shweder, 1991). From this perspective, the culture is viewed as intersubjective reality through which we know, create and experience the world we live. Different cultures are viewed as independently developing their own health care systems, such as Ayurveda, acupuncture, Unāni systems and voodoo. The third approach of indigenous psychology primarily refers to the study of tribes, aboriginals or first nations, as the term used in the West. These are the ethnic groups which are not part of the mainstream cultures. Their healing practices have been termed as magico-religious and are only recently subjected to scientific investigation (Dalal, 2011). Lo and Fung (2003) have shown that indigenous therapies are effective, and mostly as effective as the Western psychotherapies in the case of mental illnesses. Western allopathic medicine and psychotherapies, which are at present adopted by almost all countries of the world and are, in fact, examples of one kind of indigenous health care systems.

In a short span of two decades, cultural psychology of health has emerged as a serious field of research and medical training in the West (Gurung, 2014). Research publications in this area have grown exponentially and the field is open to exciting research possibilities. It is interesting to note that many alternative and complementary modes of health care are now competing with the biomedical model.

Health as Well-being

The meaning of the term health has outgrown from German and Anglo-section words implying 'whole', 'hale' and 'holy'. It thus refers to the wholesomeness of a person. Health, thus, has strong association with holiness, happiness, hygiene, cleanliness, sanity and real-self. Many of these aspects of health are emphasized in Ayurveda, Tao and Hippocratic system, which refer to health in terms of wholeness and harmony with nature. These are the primary considerations along which healing systems in traditional societies have evolved and coexist along with Western medicine in the present times. It is acknowledged in most of the traditional health care systems that there is a close symbiotic relationship between mind and body, and the goal of sound health attained by taking care of the both.

It should be clear from the above discussion that health cannot be defined within the narrow view of illness or its absence. The much publicized definition given by WHO (1978) has rightly stated health as "the state of complete physical, mental, and social well-being, and not merely an absence of disease or infirmity." This definition views health beyond the mere absence of a disease and focuses on maintaining good health, rather than on the treatment of different diseases. It takes health as a multidimensional concept—the three components of health being physical, mental and social. Health, thus, refers to proper functioning of the body and the mind, as well as, the capacity to participate in social activities, performing the roles and abiding by the moral principles. It takes into consideration the nutritional status, immunity from diseases, and better quality of social and family life. In fact, the concept of good health is considered as synonymous to the general well-being of a person. The concern is not with cure, that is, treating and preventing organic malfunctioning, but with healing the person, that is, regenerating a sense of well-being and fitness to deal with one's life conditions. Clearly, the emphasis in the WHO definition is on the positive rather than on the negative side of health.

The WHO definition has been under sustained attack almost since its inception. It is still within the extended domain of Western medicine where the emphasis is on individual well-being within the material world. The three components are viewed as distinct entities which collectively determine the health status of an individual. Importantly, the spiritual component, though included in many WHO studies, is not part of its very definition. Faith in God and supernatural are considered the aspects of any construction of health where people often attribute their good health or recovery from a major illness to the supernatural causation. In January 1998, the Executive Board of WHO adopted a resolution recommending that the World Health Assembly should add the word 'spiritual' to the definition of health. But the resolution was not adopted by the general membership at that time and is still pending.

Critics further argue that the WHO definition of health is utopian, inflexible and unrealistic, and that including the word 'complete' in the definition makes it highly unlikely that anyone would be healthy for a reasonable period of time. It also appears that 'a state of complete physical mental and social well-being' corresponds more to happiness than to health (Saracci, 1997). The words 'health' and 'happiness' designate distinct life experiences, whose relationship is neither fixed nor constant. Failure to distinguish happiness from health implies that any disturbance in happiness, however minimal, may come to be perceived as a health problem.

Health is like a dynamic field in which different elements operate in communion and harmony. A revised view of health recognizes various levels of existence in human life and progression to higher planes. Thus, a revised definition of health should read like "Health is a dynamic balance of physical, mental, social and moral modes of being aspiring for higher existence; not just the absence of evil, illness or infirmity."

The concept of health subsumes all four domains—treatment, prevention of disease, promotion of good health, and rehabilitation of mentally and physically disabled. Such a comprehensive definition brings into the fold of health care not only the medical practitioners but also counsellors, family members, community leaders and traditional practitioners. Accordingly, health can not only be studied as medical, psychological and scientific concern, but it also needs to be placed in the larger social, political and global context. This widening domain of health as well-being brings to its fold the totality of human existence and its institutional network. Consequently, the concepts of health and well-being cannot be confined within the narrow disciplinary boundaries of psychology and medicine; rather they draw from many other social as well as natural science disciplines.

Relationship between Health and Illness

All textbooks in this area treat health and illness as twin concepts; one is often defined in the context of the other. Taken together, they cover the whole spectrum of healthiness and provide a fuller understanding of the related issues. Health and illness are considered to be related to each other in three different ways. These three ways are: as opposites, as a continuum, or as different regions. Taking them as polar opposites implies that people are either healthy or unhealthy. Although to remain healthy is the cherished state, people fall ill and remain so till they are cured. This is how the medical model defines health, that is, in terms of the absence of illness. It is only when pain and other accompanying physical symptoms subside that one is again in healthy state. Medical science thus focuses on the disease, its diagnosis and treatment regimen. Defining health as opposite to illness breaks down when a person is at the same time healthy and ill. One may be suffering from a disease but may be in good spirit. Physical state is only one aspect of it, other being mental, social and moral where the dichotomy does not make much sense. As Radley (1994) noted, taking health and illness as dichotomous is a linguistic artefact.

The second view is to take health and illness along a continuum, implying that the distinction is a matter of degree only. No one is completely healthy or sick but stays somewhere along the continuum. Sometimes health and illness are taken as two separate but interdependent components, as two dimensions of health. In this, it is possible that one is on the lower side of the physical and on the higher side of the mental health continuum. A composite view is, however, considered to be providing an overall picture of health. Again, as the experiential state of health, there could be wide variations in the way people feel at different points of time. Such a continuum implies that it is possible to quantify and measure health status of a person. This view assumes that people are able to report their actual mental and physical state and the measures are psychometrically sound and valid.

The third view holds health and illness as separate, non-overlapping regions and a person belongs to either of the two regions. If we are lucky, we spend most of our time in the health region, though most of us at some point in time stay in the other region, or at the border

(Radley, 1994). People have their own beliefs about what it means to be belonging to one region and not to the other. People learn ways and means of making crossover and also of staying in the health region. This view emphasizes more on experiential and feeling aspects of health and illness. This view seems to be closer to the psychological understanding of health. According to this view, even the terminally ill patients may be happy, enjoying their remaining life.

Before we move further, it may be useful to clarify the distinction among three terms which are many times used interchangeably. These are: disease, illness and sickness. Kleinman (1980) has clarified the distinction among these terms. The term 'disease' refers to the bodily condition, some pathology and its diagnosis. Disease is something which physicians diagnose and treat. Examples include cancer, viral fever and tuberculosis, each one having its distinct symptoms. Illness refers to the experience of that disease; the way people understand their disease, respond to it and experience the bodily changes. Illness, thus, deals with as to how people experience pain and bodily changes. It can be stated here that people may feel the illness even in the absence of bodily symptoms and sometimes do not feel disease even when the symptoms are there. While watching a good movie, we forget the physical pain, but the same gets aggravated when we are in a bad mood. 'Sickness' can be defined as a social role of the diseased persons. It refers to the way in which a sick person is and should be treated by the society; how a sick person should behave. Clearly, disease is a medical term; illness refers to its psychological side and sickness refers to the sociology of the diseased person. This distinction is important to understand the distinction between health and illness.

The Biomedical Model of Medicine

The biomedical model of medicine has originated in the West, in the nineteenth century and has prospered on significant discoveries in the field of medical science. It has now attained worldwide acceptance and has been adopted as an official health care programme by almost all countries. India is no exception where official health policies and programmes have primarily relied on the biomedical model. It has almost overshadowed and replaced the Ayurvedic system of health care in India. The vast network of hospitals, dispensaries and also primary health centres is manned by the professionals trained in the biomedical tradition.

Emanating from the Cartesian dualism of mind and body as proposed by Descartes, the biomedical model considers disease as a form of biological malfunctioning—some kind of biochemical imbalance or neurophysiological disturbance. In this, the body is held as a machine that can be examined in terms of its parts, that is, as a system of synchronized organs. A disease is seen as impaired functioning of a biological mechanism and the doctor's role is to intervene, either physically or chemically, the malfunctioning of the specific body part (Capra, 1983). In this biomedical model, psychological and social processes are considered to be independent of the disease process. Though the emotional state of the patient is considered important, it is kept outside the purview of medical treatment.

The biomedical theory of disease grew around the conviction that most diseases are caused by invaders from the outside 'micro-organisms or germs'. It is believed that there is one causal or contributing factor, some outside organism, which is responsible for the disease, and there can be one specific biological (chemical) solution of the problem. The discovery of antibiotics in the 1930s and 1940s gave impetus to the modern medicine; the 'miracle drugs' seized public imagination. There were great hopes that medical science would eventually discover an effective drug therapy to eradicate every known disease; that, there will be 'a pill for every ill'. This belief was so strong that even emotional and mental disorders were treated with various drugs, ignoring their psychogenic antecedents. The biomedical model of health care has not fulfilled the expectations it aroused. Adherence to this model has helped in reducing mortality by controlling the prevalence of contagious diseases. The human life span is increasing all over the world though the actual contribution of biomedicine towards this success is debated. Improved economic status, social hygiene and health consciousness have also made a significant difference in this scenario (Taylor, 2006). Moreover, though the rate of mortality is going down, an increasingly large population continues to suffer from various chronic and degenerative diseases.

The biomedical model has many serious limitations (Bhugra & Bhui, 2007). The model treats a patient as an organism, a biological entity. The proponents of this model were more interested in the disease than the patient. Thus, when the curative aspect is taken up, the emphasis is on the nature of diseases, its various symptoms and on the ways to remove them. In this process, the patient is only a recipient of certain medication, and no cognizance is taken of the psychological state of the patient. Biomedical practices envisage no role for the patient and his or her support group in the process of diagnosis and in deciding about the course of treatment. The interest in the patient as a person is only incidental. As Siegel (1986, p. 2) has rightly observed, "[medical] practitioners still act as though disease catches people, rather than understanding that people catch disease by becoming susceptible to the germs of the illness to which we are constantly exposed."

Thus, most of the health schemes focus on providing better medical facilities rather than involving the patient towards a common goal of attending to the sickness. Quite often medical practitioners learn from their personal experiences that diagnosis would be more accurate and treatment more effective if patient's socio-economic and cultural background, beliefs, needs and anxieties are also taken into consideration. Nevertheless, it is presumed that the patient would be receptive, willing to supply all necessary information and would conform to the treatment regimen. This may be so, at the most, in the case of hospitalized patients. In cases of chronic diseases, patients and their families do not always accept the passive role and frequently engage in their own, at times, "in some secret forms of curing," depending on their appraisal of the disease and its future course (Engel, 1977). The biomedical model views the practices of faith and spiritual healing with scepticism, and with that, cultural traditions of managing health problems are undermined.

The biomedical model played a major role in eradicating many diseases which had killed millions of people during the 1920s–1930s. Penicillin and sulpha drugs were held as miracle drugs all over to save people from epidemics. Many of life-threatening and disabling diseases are now completely eradicated. In the present time, however, the efficacy of biomedical model is seriously questioned in the case of preventive health care. In this case, there are no cooperative, captive patients, where people are under no compulsion to comply with the prescribed health procedures. People may ignore, or may pay little attention when they are told about the adverse health consequences of some of their own habits, like smoking. There are also differences in the meaning of illness and health in different cultures and in the threat perception of various diseases. Promotion of good health is again beyond the scope of the biomedical model.

Psychosomatic Illness

The existing medical practices have, in reality, not completely ignored the psychological basis of many diseases such as ulcers, coronary heart diseases, bronchitis and hypertension. The causal connection between mental disorders and physical diseases is a subject of serious discussion within biomedical sciences. The diseases which have psychogenic base are called psychosomatic diseases. This branch of medicine, though, acknowledges that many diseases are caused by psychological factors, yet no distinction is made in terms of treatment.

Psychological stress is considered to be the main cause of psychosomatic diseases. What does a stressful life event do to a person? Selye (1976) has argued for a three-phase reaction to psychological stress. First is the alarm phase, during which people mobilize all their social and psychological resources to combat the threat. In the second phase, people make efforts to cope with the threat, as through confrontation. In the third phase, exhaustion occurs if people fail to overcome the threat and deplete their physical resources. This could lead to the onset of physical symptoms. Much depends on how an individual appraises the stressors, and on the social support and intrapersonal resources available to a person (Lazarus, 1966; Mason, 1971). In their later work, Lazarus and Folkman (1984) showed much interest in cataclysmic events which have sudden and powerful impact and which are more or less universal in eliciting a response. Events like natural disaster (flood and cyclone), accidents, life-threatening diseases (heart disease, cancer and AIDS) are unpredictable and serious threats. Coping in such cases is long term and there may be no immediate recovery. People show all kinds of physical symptoms while going through such life crisis.

The Second World War caused immense human tragedies, resulting in the study and treatment of the effects of psychological traumas on physical health. In a large number of hospitals, separate departments of 'psychosomatic medicine' were started. These departments aimed to understand, for example, how episodes of anger and hostility can translate into stomach ulcers and heart attacks. But, because medicine so rigidly compartmentalized the realms of mind and body, this new discipline never got the respect it deserved (Benson, 1997). In the long run, this may have been for the best as, obviously, no one discipline can address the complex interrelatedness of the mind and the body.

Subsequently, in clinical practices, both in medical and clinical psychology, the classification of diseases as 'psychosomatic' was seriously questioned; so much so that in DSM-4-TR (as brought out by the American Psychological Association, 2004), the category of psychosomatic diseases has been eliminated. The latest version DSM-5 (2013) has again added up many new categories of mental problems which border on psychosomatic illnesses.

Health and Well-being in Indian Culture

The term parallel to health in the Sanskrit language is *swastha*, literally meaning 'that which is situated in own-self'. Monier-Williams Dictionary (revised, 2008) termed swastha as 'being in one's self', 'being in one's natural state', 'relying upon one's self' and 'self-sufficient'. Health thus means the state of being, located inside the self. It is the inner state not contingent on nutritional, physical and material factors but on individual's entire existential condition.

The conceptualization of the state of well-being is closer to the concept of mental health and happiness, life satisfaction and actualization of one's full potential. Verma and Verma (1989) have defined 'general well-being' as the subjective feeling of contentment, happiness, satisfaction with life experiences and of one's role in the world of work, sense of achievement, utility, belongingness, and no distress, dissatisfaction or worry. This conception of subjective well-being is much inspired by the work of Diener and his group (Diener, 1984, 2000; Diener, Oishi & Lucas, 2003).

In the traditional Indian conceptualization, health is conceived in a wider sense of total well-being and happiness (Sinha, 1990). It is the absence of not only pain and suffering but also in terms of many positive dispositions. It included the cultivation of many personality attributes, emotional state, intellectual capacities and moral values, such as inner peace, truthfulness and self-knowledge. A person who is detached and equipoised in pain and pleasure is considered in the highest state of well-being. As Sinha noted, in Indian tradition, this state of well-being and happiness is contingent on happiness and health of all other living beings and that no one wishes unhappiness to anyone.[1] Health and well-being are thus presumed to be contingent not only on the state of one's own self, but also on the state of other's selves, which includes all living creatures.

In the Indian tradition, health and well-being are understood not only in terms of human body and its functions but also in terms of mental status and supernatural aspects (Salagame, 2013). The unhealthy state is understood more in terms of suffering. A person going through prolonged illness may be suffering due to physical pain and discomfort, and/or uncertainty, loneliness, family crisis, and/or guilt or supernatural considerations. The Indian notion of a healthy person is of an auto-locus person (swastha) who flourishes on the recognition of life force derived from the material reality (*mahābhutas*) and, therefore, offers remedies for being healthy by opening a dialogue with its environment and observing one's duty (dharma). The nutrition (*ahar*), world of leisure (*vihar*) and thoughts (*vichar*) need to be synchronized in proper order. Health and well-being are both personal as well as social. The desire for the well-being of everyone (*Kamayé duhkhtaptanam praninamartinshanam*) has been a core Indian concern that has panhuman relevance. Undoubtedly, such a conceptualization of health and well-being is significant to study in the larger perspective (Sharma & Misra, 2009), in which physical, metaphysical and supernatural are part of the larger reality.

Ayurvedic Model of Health

The term Ayurveda literary means 'a science of life and longevity' (*āyus* means 'life, vitality, health, longevity', and *veda* means 'science or knowledge'). Ayurveda offers an approach to health care that aims to achieve longevity and health ageing (Manohar, 2013). This system of medicine offers a different perspective on life and health, in which wholeness, integration, freedom, connectivity, creativity and enjoyment figure as central concerns. It is the ancient medical system of India being practised for more than 3,000 years. The authorship of the most basic text of Ayurveda is attributed to Charaka, who essentially compiled the proceedings of a conference, known as the *Charaka Samhitā*.

---

[1] *Sarvey bhavantu sukhinah sarve santu nirāmayah, Sarve bhādrani pāshyantu mā kashchid dukhābhag bhavet.*

Ayurvedic medicine was already well developed by the time of Buddha. The famous Indian universities of that period, Nalanda and Taxashila produced many great physicians.

According to Ayurveda, any disturbance, physical or mental, manifests itself both in the somatic and in the psychic spheres, through the intermediary process of the vitiation of the 'humors'. Ayurvedic therapy aims at correcting the *doshas* or the imbalances and derangements of the bodily humors (namely *vāta* or bodily air, *pitta* or bile and *kapha* or phlegm) and restoring equilibrium. As Fields (2001, p. 52) has articulated,

> healing involves restoration of balanced states of being within the organism—that is, at the level of the doshas or constituent principles of the mind/body complex, and between organism and environment. Broadly conceived, equilibrium in Āyurveda means the stable and harmonious functioning of our organs and systems, psyche and spirit, but also, a balanced and creative relationship with our fellow creatures and nature as a whole.

It does so by coordinating all of the material, mental and spiritual resources of the whole person, recognizing that the essence of these potencies is the manifestation of cosmic forces. In principle, Ayurvedic therapy for all diseases cannot be other than a blend of the psychological and the physiological. In practice, the psychological part of the treatment comprises suggestion, exhortation, consolation and recommendation of meditative procedures. Even for diseases of primarily mental origins and with predominantly mental symptoms, it is overwhelmingly a psychological therapy for the psyche. There are three therapies with regard to their location of action: 'scientific' therapy, which uses proper diet, activities and remedies according to season and climate, at the level of the physical body; 'mind therapy' involving restraint of the mind from the desire for unwholesome objects; and 'divine' therapy, including all sorts of spiritual rituals and penance. Medical intervention at the physical level is of four types: diet, activity, purification and palliation (Svoboda, 1992). In his treatise *Ayurveda and Modern Medicine*, Lele (1986) has elaborated on ontology, theory and practices of Ayurveda as a well-evolved science of living and well-being.

As Kakar (1982) has posited, Ayurveda is a principal architect of the Indian concepts of person and the body. As a paradigm, it shows how body, mind and spirit interactions can be predicted, balanced and improved upon to enable people to live gracefully and harmoniously. For Ayurveda, spirit and matter, soul and body, although different, are not alien, insofar as they can be brought together in a healthy relationship with consequences that are mutually beneficial. Its prime concern is not with 'healing' in the narrow sense of curing illness but in the broader sense of promoting health and well-being and prolonging life. The goal of this enhanced vitality is the achievement of all the values that life has to offer, both secular and religious. In Ayurveda, balance or equilibrium (*sama*) is synonymous with health. Also, the maintenance of equilibrium is health and, conversely, the disturbance of the equilibrium of tissue elements characterizes the state of disease. The person in Ayurveda is conceived of as simultaneously living in and partaking of different orders of being—physical, social and spiritual. Inclusion of spirituality as a fourth dimension, in addition to the three dimensions of physical, mental and social, vitalizes the other three aspects. It may be noted that the boundaries between these levels are fluid as they are interconnected and complement to each other.

There are no general prescriptions in Ayurvedic treatment for different diseases; rather, it is tailor-made for each person depending on his/her physical and mental constitution. Every person is presumed to be a complex and unique expression of their physical and mental make-up (Manohar, 2013). The constitution of the individual is considered to be setting limits and possibilities for the person to attain a certain level of health status. A physician's personality and attitude is considered crucial in the recovery of the patient in Ayurveda. Lele (1986) stated that an Ayurvedic physician is supposed to have the same attributes as mentioned in the most popular textbook of internal medicine by Harrison— tact, sympathy and understanding.

Ayurveda remains a living tradition, a way of living. For centuries, Ayurveda has guided the lifestyle of people and help organizing the practices of daily living, including food preferences, leisure activities, and preventive and promotive health measures in India (Chopra, 1990). The knowledge of Ayurvedic medicines has flown from the guru to the disciple. Though in reality, as many studies have shown, professionalized Ayurvedic doctors have become wholly body-oriented, unlike the traditional *vaidyas*, who are still holistic in their orientation. Svoboda (1992) stated that as long as Ayurveda remains a way of life as a universal art of healing, it will always exist and pervade individual consciousness.

Other Health Systems in India

In addition to Ayurveda, India has a whole range of other medicinal and curative systems dealing with a wide range of health problems. These alternative systems have been providing services for centuries in different parts of the country and are thriving on the popular public support in the recent times as well. Some of these popular systems are included in the public health care programmes of the government. In fact, the Central Government has established a separate Department of AYUSH (Ayurveda, Yoga, Unāni, Siddha and Homeopathy) within the Ministry of Health to promote practice and research in some prominent alternative systems of health care.

Health and Well-being: A Schematic Model

Dalal and Misra (2006) proposed this comprehensive model of health and well-being which includes the whole gamut of psychosocial conditions which are linked with health, as causes, concomitants and consequences. This schematic model is presented in Figure 1.1.

This model builds on the three main domains of health conceived as: 'restoration, maintenance and growth' of life processes. The first domain is essentially that of illness where the primary focus is on bringing the person back from the state of illness (incongruity/disjunction) to the state of health or re-establishing the congruence and conjunction. Here, health practically implies the process of recovery from the disease. Thus, it involves curative and healing interventions that can free the patient from the bodily suffering and pain. Patients, health practitioners, caregivers and hospitals are part of this domain. Disability rehabilitation also falls within it.

The second domain of health is that of maintenance, which has been until recently ignored by all stakeholders. The major concern in this domain is to engage in the activities to maintain good health and protect oneself from diseases and disabilities. Health is not static or fixed. It's a dynamic process and one's present health status is no guarantee that it will remain the same in future. People who primarily belong to this domain take charge of their health. They have to be motivated to act proactively to enhance their immunity, resistance to diseases, resilience,

Figure 1.1:
Domains of health: Restoration, maintenance and growth

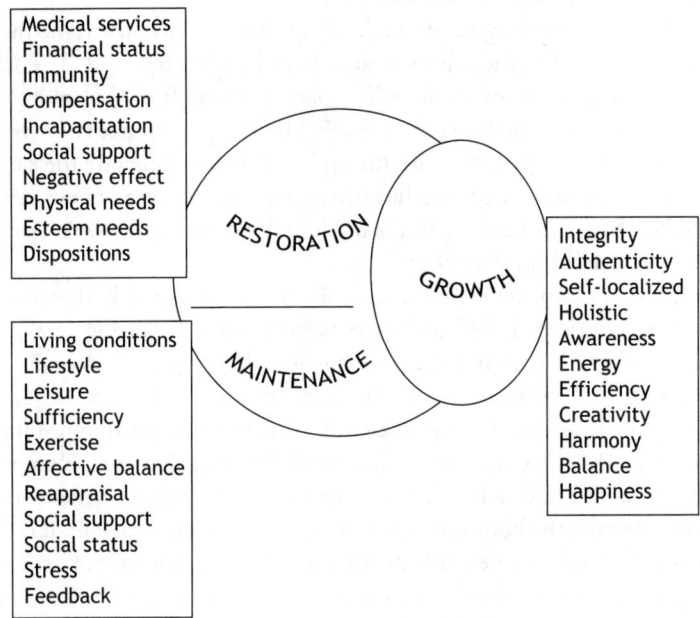

Medical services
Financial status
Immunity
Compensation
Incapacitation
Social support
Negative effect
Physical needs
Esteem needs
Dispositions

Living conditions
Lifestyle
Leisure
Sufficiency
Exercise
Affective balance
Reappraisal
Social support
Social status
Stress
Feedback

RESTORATION

MAINTENANCE

GROWTH

Integrity
Authenticity
Self-localized
Holistic
Awareness
Energy
Efficiency
Creativity
Harmony
Balance
Happiness

Source: Dalal and Misra (2011).

physical and mental vitality, and active participation in family and communal lives. In other words, this domain involves the personal as well as social or relational space. On the one hand, the person has to perform exercise and yoga, do work and take proper diet; on the other, he or she has to be active in continuing and nourishing the social relations with family, co-workers and environment.

The third health domain is of growth orientation. It can be referred to as psycho-spiritual health. The person evolves and goes beyond the isolated and limited self. In this domain, health is seen from a much wider perspective that encompasses holistic (physical, social and spiritual) existence of a person. The awareness or consciousness of a person is to be established in both the physical and moral or ethical spaces. The person strives to achieve a level of functioning that ensures enfoldment of human potential to grow and realize one's life goals. The blossoming of inherent potential may also result in efficiency, energy and creativity. A journey which may begin with restoration from disease (*vyadhi*) may thus continue towards the state of self-realization, equanimity and calmness, in sum, towards blissful existence.

There is, in fact, a great deal of overlap and permeability in the three domains of health, though these are hierarchically organized. The salience of these domains in one's life space keeps shifting (shrinking or expanding). The relative space occupied by the growth domain would determine one's quality of health and well-being. Second, the antecedents and consequents are linearly arrayed in the case of restorative health, where the main interest is in identifying the factors which cause the disease and lead to recovery.

As posited, in maintenance domain, the causality is bidirectional. In that, emotions, beliefs and expectations play a balancing role, and are both—the causes and the consequences. In the growth domain, an individual can create and control these psychological factors so as to deploy them for performing efficiently. Third, the interaction of mind, body and self is a crucial condition in all the three domains. However, whereas in the restoration domain, the emphasis is more on the mental states affecting the body condition, in the maintenance domain, it is the harmonious relation between the two which is of prime importance; in the growth domain, the focus is on psychological factors and a harmonious relation among mind–body–soul (self).

Psychosocial Factors in Health and Well-being

A large body of research has accumulated to substantiate the argument advanced in the above model that the psychological factors affect the physical health. A variety of psychological factors including personal dispositions, moods states, attitudes, beliefs, expectations and affective states are documented as both causes and concomitants of one's health and well-being.

Chronic Stress and Immune System

Tragic and undesirable life events which cause stress over a long period of time are found to be adversely affecting physical health of a person. There is a body of research evidence that grief, depression and other negative feelings are linked with the increased risk of organic (like cancer) and infectious (like cold) diseases. For example, recent bereavement has been linked with the increased risk of a number of diseases, such as coronary heart disease, tuberculosis, allergies and peptic ulcers (Taylor, 2006). Stress-related negative emotions tend to suppress body's immune system over an extended time, rendering the person vulnerable to a host of diseases.

The immune system protects the body from the invading microorganisms—bacteria, virus, fungi and parasites. These are called antigens. The immune system of the body, rather than being a centralized system, operates through a blood circulatory process throughout the body and gets activated wherever antigens are encountered, called lymphocytes, these are special types of white blood cells, medically called T-cells, B-cells and NK (natural killer)-cells. These blood cells multiply, differentiate and mature in the bone marrow, thymus, lymph nodes and spleen and in other body parts. The lymphocytes produce their own antigens to mobilize a direct attack to kill the invading foreign microorganisms in the blood stream. Glasser (1976) pointed out that the immune system must be extraordinarily efficient in destroying the invading bacteria and viruses on an ongoing basis to keep us healthy. Even when they temporarily give in, they always keep the fight going on. It is only when the body's immune system is destroyed by a virus called Human Immuno-deficiency Virus (HIV) that people become highly vulnerable to all kinds of infections.

In recent years, a new field of psychoimmunoneurology has emerged to examine the mediating role of psychological factors in immune deficiency. The body's immune system is presumed to be interacting with the central nervous system and endocrine system, on one hand, and with the psychological and social aspects of life, on the other. Vaillant and Mukamal (2001) have discussed involuntary mental mechanisms that adaptively alter the inner and/or outer reality to minimize the level of stress. More chronic the stress is, more severe is the damage caused to the immune system. Kiecolt-Glaser, Speicher, Holliday and Glaser (1984) found that examination stress results in poorer immunocompetence, more so for the lonely students. Kiecolt-Glaser, Fisher, Ogrock, Stout, Speicher and Glaser (1997) found that women who were recently separated had lower immunity than married women.

The effect of chronic stress on the body's immune functioning is, however, mediated by a number of factors, including nature and severity of stressors. For example, the stressors which are uncontrollable produce more adverse effects than those which are controllable. Again, people who were more depressed were found to be more susceptible to infectious diseases and had slower recovery rate. Schleifer, Eckholdt, Cohen and Keller (1993) and Schleifer, Keller, Bond, Cohen and Stein (1989) discovered on the basis of empirical work and meta-analysis that depression was associated with immunodepression, primarily among older and hospitalized patients. Also, a mild physical stress experienced in the recent past was sufficient enough to enhance immunity against the adverse effects of the present stress experience. In a meta-analytic study conducted on 293 articles published between 1960 and 2001, Segerstrom and Miller (2004) confirmed that chronic stress suppresses body's immune system, while short-term stress enhances it.

However, not much is still known about the possible physical mechanism through which psychosocial factors operate and play an important role. Several lines of work suggest that psychosocial stress alters the composition of brain chemicals, triggering chain reactions in the central nervous system and the hypothalamus, which regulates the secretions of the endocrine system and increase the level of corticoid in the blood. The corticoid in the blood is presumed to damage lymphocytes and lower the efficiency of the immune system. Chronic stresses, negative emotions and lack of social support often silently block the breeding of NK-cells in the blood stream. The stress exposure can cause the glucocorticoid hormone to be overly active which causes a depletion of norepinephrine levels in locus coeruleus neurons. It has an effect of slowing the attentiveness and physical alertness within the individual (Salzano, 2003). These findings are, however, suggestive of the possible linkages and could be mediated by a large number of concomitant factors.

Individual Dispositions and Life-threatening Diseases

Many individual dispositions were also found to have significant bearings on health status. There are personality traits that predispose an individual to a negative emotional state, such as depression, anxiety and nervousness, or leads to maladaptive coping behaviours. Mathews and Ridgeway (1981) identified a large number of personality variables associated with surgical recovery. Feelings of control and positive attitude were found to be important factors in the success of surgery (Hunt, McKenna, Backett & Pope, 1984). Also, recovery from major surgery was found to be contingent on patient's emotional state prior to the surgery (see Cohen & Lazarus, 1979; Mason, 1971). Janis (1958) found a curvilinear relationship between anticipatory fear and post-operative recovery. Sartorius (2002) contended that physical health and mental health are closely associated through various mechanisms, as studies of the links between depression and heart and vascular disease are demonstrating.

A well-known personality disposition is Type A behaviour pattern that significantly contributes to the occurrence of coronary heart disease (Glass, 1976; Jenkins, 1974). A Type A person shows extreme competitiveness, a sense of urgency (always feels rushed or is impatient when delayed), excessive involvement in work, aggressiveness and hostility. Individuals displaying this behaviour pattern seem to be engaged in chronic, ceaseless and unnecessary struggle with themselves, with others and with circumstances. In contrast, Type B behaviour pattern is characterized by a low level of competitiveness, time urgency and hostility. They are easy-going and philosophical.

In a study of eight and a half year follow-up of more than 5,000 people, Rosenman and others (1970) confirmed that Type A behaviour is strongly related to coronary heart disease incidences. The mortality from this disease was twice as high in Type A patients than in Type B patients. Their study revealed that those who exhibited competitive lifestyle were more likely to develop coronary heart disease (myocardial infarction, angina pectoris and silent heart attack) even when biological risk factors (like smoking) were controlled. Weiss and Lonnquist (1996) suggested three possible mediators between Type A behaviour and heart disease—(a) some underlying physical weakness may be associated with Type A behaviour, (b) hyper-responsivity of Type A person may cause over-activity of sympathetic nervous system (SNS) and (c) Type A behaviour leads to more risky circumstances, such as delay in treatment. However, some studies (Gallacher, Sweetnam, Yarnell, Elwood & Stansfeld, 2003) found both confirmatory and null results taking Type A behaviour pattern. Many Indian studies (Dalal, 2012) have also confirmed that Type A people are more prone to heart problems than their Type B counterparts.

A similar search for a cancer-prone personality has also not been very successful. There is some evidence that those who develop cancer are unable to express positive feelings, make an extensive use of repressive measures and make less use of ego defence (Eyenck, 1988). Longer survival rate among cancer patients was associated with more frequent expression of hostility and other negative feelings (Derogatis, Abeloff & Melisaratos, 1979). A different personality pattern, known as Type C personality, has been identified, which is cancer prone. Psychologists have now identified a 'Type C' (cancer-prone) personality as the one that responds to stress with depression and with a sense of hopelessness. Type C personalities have a tendency to be introvert, respectful, eager to please, conforming and compliant. Type C people are basically nice guys who never show anger and other negative reactions in public. They are helping and cooperative and they smile and never hurt others, but at the same time, they never express their true feelings. These are lonely people, even shy of seeking help when need be. Derogatis discovered that Type C people have four times higher risk of cancer than others. However, most of the recent studies show small and inconsistent relationships between personality, immunity and cancer that have led some to question whether these relationships are important (Sagerstrom, 2003).

Still another personality pattern, termed as Type D personality was reported to be closely linked with a high rate of mortality by Denollet (2000). According to Denollet (2000, 2004), Type D personality comprises two broad and stable traits: (a) negative affectivity—people who have greater tendency to experience negative feelings. People high on this trait often feel unhappy, tend to worry, are depressed, easily irritable, and lack self-esteem and assertiveness; (b) social inhibition—tendency to inhibit feelings and behaviour in social situation. Such people are reserved, lack social support and avoid intimacy (Pederson, Ong, Sonnenschein, Serruys, Erdman & van Domburg, 2006). Denollet (2004) predicted that such personality may aggravate disease directly through pathophysiological mechanism. It is quite likely that Type D personality may precipitate heart attack, as well as many other fatal diseases.

Cognitive Orientation and Health Risk

As stated by Lazarus (1984), people construe a stressful life event in their own idiosyncratic ways. Many studies have focused on the manner in which people appraise the severity of life events, their causal explanations and ramifications. Some people are more negative in their subjective construction of an event, view the situation as uncontrollable and feel helpless and hopeless. Abramson, Seligman and Teasdale (1978) postulated a pessimistic explanatory style, characterized by internal (self), stable and global explanations of the negative events. The pessimistic explanatory style and depression have been found to be positively related. In a 35-year longitudinal study, Peterson, Seligman and Valliant (1988) found that pessimistic explanatory style was not linked with poor health at the age of 25, but significantly predicted poor health above the age of 45 years. One explanation was that at a young age, people have physical resources to absorb negativity, but these get depleted as their age advances. A prospective study of coronary heart disease (CHD) and optimism found that "a more optimistic explanatory style, or viewing the glass as half full, lowers the risk of CHD in older men" (Kubzansky, Sparrow, Vokonas & Kawachi, 2001: 911, 913) and discussed other research showing a link "between pessimism, hopelessness, and risk of heart disease." Agarwal and Dalal (1993) found that beliefs in the doctrine of karma and God, which give rise to hope, facilitated recovery from myocardial infarction. Solberg and Segerstrom (2006) examined in their meta-analysis the relationship between optimism and coping crossed optimistic and pessimistic styles, fitting coping responses from various studies into four categories. Optimism was positively associated with broad measures of engagement coping and problem-focused coping.

Positive orientation or thinking about the crisis is another important cognition that has wide implications for recovery from any disease. Studies (Scheier & Carver, 1985; Scheier, Weintraub & Carver, 1986) have shown that optimism (generalized expectancy of good outcomes) is associated with problem-focused coping, seeking social support, seeing the positive side of the illness and acceptance of uncontrollable outcomes. Taylor (1983) observed that positive comparison was often used by cancer patients for self-enhancement in the event of an accident or illness. The patients who compared themselves with those who were in worse conditions recovered earlier. In a study by Agrawal, Dalal, Agrawal and Agrawal (1994), positive life orientation emerged as an important predictor of medical, as well as of psychological recovery of myocardial patients. In a comprehensive review study, Rasmussen, Scheier and Greenhouse (2009) stated that optimists may be less reactive than pessimists to the stresses of life; the lower physiological stress responses may (over many years) result in less physical wear and tear on the body; the end result may be better physical health and even greater longevity.

Health-impairing Behaviour

In general, behavioural factors exert influence on health and illness of people in four ways: health enhancing, health impairing, health protective and illness management. Diet, exercise and meditation are health-enhancing behaviours; tobacco chewing and alcoholism will come under health-impairing behaviours. The examples of health protective behaviours are immunization, maintaining hygiene and pollution-free environment, whereas illness management refers to taking initiatives to recover from an impending illness. Here, we may focus more on the behaviours which have adverse consequences on health; directly or indirectly they become causative factors in the onset of a disease.

Much of the Western literature in dealing with health-impairing behaviours has focused on smoking, on obesity and to a lesser extent on alcoholism. What people eat and how much they weigh are considered behavioural processes which in concert with genetic and metabolic characteristics shape the health of a person (Baum & Posluszny, 1999). An unhealthy diet appears to directly enhance the risk of a disease, as low level of nutrition may contribute to pathophysiology of disease, as tobacco chewing, smoking, drug use and alcohol consumption may have direct effects on bodily systems and impair their efficiency. In low-income countries like India, under-nutrition and malnutrition becomes a major risk factor.

Consumption of tobacco in different forms is pervasive all over the world. Once tobacco use becomes a habit, it is highly resistant to change. The primary active ingredient in tobacco is nicotine, which has stimulant properties that increases SNS arousal, alertness and reduces appetite. Smoking and other forms of tobacco use are major contributors to heart diseases, hypertension, stroke, cancer and other diseases. Passive exposure to tobacco smoke is also problematic and has similar effects as that of smoking. Consumption of tobacco in different forms is very common in India and has been found to be significantly associated with cancer.

Alcoholism, drugs and other narcotics are no lesser evil and are much more rampant than smoking. In India, about 3 million consume various narcotics, mostly heroin and brown sugar (Pant & Bagrodia, 2003). In the case of alcoholism, it is suggested in many studies that it is not alcohol consumption per se which affect health but the pattern of drinking, rather its abuse. Moderate level of drinking is considered to be good for health in many Western studies. Alcohol consumption becomes a health hazard when it is used as a mechanism for stress alleviation. Its association with social and moral aspects of behaviour often poses serious health problems at individual and family levels.

Stress is supposed to affect diet and weight in many ways. People who are under stress or in negative mood state are often seen eating more. They seek, what is called 'comfort foods' or foods that make them feel better. Most of these foods are relatively high in fat and salt or sugar, meaning that stress may increase consumption of less healthy food. Such people gain weight and loose stamina to fight stress. In some cases, increased metabolic demand during stress may increase consumption of food without necessarily affecting weight. The growing craze for fast and junk food and synthetic drinks is becoming a serious health hazard for the teenagers. Obesity has become a major problem in all countries. In the United States, obesity is declared a disability within the Americans with Disability Act. According to Price and Pecjak (2003), women, particularly, are more affected by the stigma of obesity because they are judged more on the basis of appearance than men.

Obesity and weight gain is a problem for a section of the society, whereas a much larger section of the society which is below poverty line suffers from malnutrition. While good nutrition enables one to lead a socially and economically active life, malnutrition has an adverse impact on health and life expectancy and increases the mortality rate. It retards physical growth, leads to functional impairment, disability and diminished productivity and reduces resistance to disease. People who are most vulnerable to malnutrition are those below poverty line and the socially disadvantaged, infants, pre-school children and pregnant women. The problem of malnutrition is a resultant of unavailability of food, low purchasing power of the people and population growth.

Under poverty conditions, women are often more malnourished. Studies have shown that in India diets of girl children and women are inadequate due to discriminatory practices. Women are discriminated in terms of both quantity and quality of the food available to them.

The low dietary intake and maternal malnutrition is a major cause of low birth weight children. Malnutrition of the mothers again causes child mortality and mental retardation in developing countries. Low status of women in the society and social practices are greatly responsible for this sorry state of affairs.

Exercise, on the contrary, is related to promoting positive health. Physical exercises play important role in managing weight, stress, as well as, in keeping oneself physically and mentally fit. Although heavy exercises adversely affect health, moderate and regular exercises keep a person physically and mentally fit.

Two kinds of physical exercises essential for good health are stretching exercises, such as Yogic asanas and aerobic exercises, such as jogging, swimming and bicycling. These exercises produce different effects and are equally essential for a healthy living. Whereas stretching exercises have a calming effect, aerobic exercises increase arousal level of the body. Yogic asanas provide systematic stretching to all the muscles and joints of the body and massages the glands and other body organs. They relax muscles and decrease their activity level. Aerobic exercises have activating and stimulating functions—to energize heart, lungs and muscles. These exercises increase heart rate and breathing and reduce the cholesterol level.

Health and Social Support

The notion of social support in health psychology is conceptualized as including both social embeddedness and emotional support that informs the people suffering from diseases that they are valued and cared about (Cobb, 1976). Social support, either elicited or provided spontaneously, goes a long way in determining how people deal with the life challenges and threats. Supportive interactions and the presence of supportive relationships in people's lives have been shown to play a major role in emotional well-being and physical health. Mother Teresa said it best: "Being unwanted is the worst disease that any human being can ever experience" (as quoted in Muggeridge, 1997: 17). Although supportive ties may create dilemmas for both the providers as well as the recipients of social support, belongingness to a reliable support system of kin and friends often reduces the risk of disease and enhances the recovery from mental and physical illness (Uchino, Uno & Holt-Lunstad, 1999).

Family as a support system has been specifically analyzed by Sharma (1999). There are two major mechanisms that explain how social support reduces the negative impact of stress on health and well-being, that is, 'direct—effects hypothesis and buffering—effect hypothesis'. Moreover, the efficacy of social support is likely to be dependent on (a) who is providing the support, (b) what kind of support is provided, (c) to whom is the support provided, (d) for what problem is the support provided and (e) when and for how long is the support provided (see Sharma, 1999). Such issues are partly reflected in a recent study by Miltiades (2002) where the effect on the psychological well-being of India-based parents was examined whose adult children had migrated to the United States. It was seen that the availability of alternative support systems (the extended family support, the hired help) did not alleviate the feelings of 'loss', depression and loneliness in such parents. Two Indian studies (Bhattacharyya, 2001; Gupta, Shama, Narayan & Gupta, 2002) did not find a direct relationship between social support and CHD. The appropriateness of a special kind of support seems to be dependent on the match between the type of support and the nature of problem encountered at a point in the life course, and also who is the provider of that support.

Psychomedical Model of Health Care

As mentioned earlier, an alternative to the biomedical model of health care, Engel (1977) introduced the biopsychosocial model to incorporate psychological and social factors in health care. For almost four decades, this reformulated model remained the basis for new subject field of health psychology. This model was essentially an extension of medical model, particularly a response to the crisis in psychiatry (Marks, 2002). The biopsychosocial model contends that health and illnesses are not just a consequence of the activities of brain and nervous system and also of psychological and cultural variables. The pre-eminence of biological factors still remains. As Armstrong (1987) observed that the theoretical basis of this model was never worked out, nor was it seriously debated. This model was largely ignored by health psychologists in recent years and virtually had no role in phenomenal progress of the field of health psychology.

In the recent writings of this author, an alternative to the biopsychosocial model is proposed. This proposed psychomedical model of health care (Dalal, 2013, 2015) which emphasizes preponderance of psychological factors over biological, in causing diseases and maintaining good health. In this respect, social, cultural and spiritual are considered as part of the mental state and consciousness of a person. In the last three decades, a host of psychological factors has come to be identified as the causes of a wide range of physical diseases and disabilities. For example, Type A personality (a person showing the characteristics of impatient, ambitious, impersonal and so on) is considered a major risk factor in CHD. Prolonged psychological stress is found to be responsible for hypertension, peptic ulcer and many other diseases. Again, psychological factors have been found important in the recovery from the physical ailments. The role of psychologists is now well recognized in the treatment of organic diseases. Patient compliance, doctor–patient communication, attitude change, self-care and so on are some of the potential areas to which health psychologists are making important contributions. Psychological factors are also important in devising strategies for health promotion and making preventive health measures more effective. Psychological rehabilitation of patients with chronic diseases and disabilities is another field that is gaining popularity.

With the increasing failure of the biomedical system in meeting health needs and alleviating human suffering, the search for alternative models of health is continuing (Wade, 2004). The emerging psychomedical approach has aroused hopes of providing better health care services. In this alternative approach, efforts are made to integrate social and psychological aspects of the illness into medical practices. For this, health psychologists are expected to team up with medical practitioners to prevent diseases and in planning the course of treatment. With vast differences in their training and orientation, such teaming up of health psychologists and physicians rarely work. Thus, though the psychomedical model was initially formulated to promote recovery of the hospital patients, it in practice never materialized.

The proposed psychomedical model emphasizes the unity of psychological factors and holistic health. In a broader sense, psychological factors influence promotional, preventive, curative and rehabilitative aspects of health. In the specific context of physical illness, this approach acknowledges that emotional and mental states affect a person's immunity to diseases and pace of recovery when they fall sick. There is a recursive causal linkage between the psychological and biological state of a person. Consequently, the recovery process is considered incomplete until one has recovered both psychologically and physically.

Bringing a person back to good health not only entails recovery from the illness but also amounts to restoring a balance of physical, social and psychological aspects within the person. This restored balance state may not necessarily be the same as the earlier one. A disease from which a person suffers is always a learning experience and it may result in a higher state of balance in which new aspects are added. The person may acquire resilience to handle a poor health condition in a more efficient way, as may be required in the case of a chronic disease. In such a case, a person may learn to balance an illness condition by cultivating a positive mental attitude and better social support so that the overall state of well-being is maintained.

Of course, this balance is dynamic and not a static one. An unstable balance in many cases may result in worsening of health condition. An individual has the ability to adapt to environmental changes and propensity to re-establish oneself in a balanced state when it is disturbed. From the psychomedical point of view, health is seen as an experience of well-being resulting from a dynamic balance that involves the physical and psychological aspects of the organism, as well as its interaction with its natural and social environment.

This new approach views a patient as a person embedded in a socio-cultural context in which he or she imbibes a certain belief system (Dalal & Ray, 2005). These socio-cultural beliefs would determine the way a patient evaluates and gives meaning to his sickness. Kleinman has made a distinction in his research between disease and illness (Kleinman, 1980). Disease is an organic malfunctioning as diagnosed by a medical practitioner, whereas illness is a subjective construction of the experience of a disease by the patient. It is a patient's own interpretation and perception of the disease, which is greatly influenced by the culture to which the patient belongs. In a traditional society like India, an illness is a social event, which concerns not only the patient but also his or her family, friends, relations and others in the social network. Everyone joins in appraising the illness.

Patients' phenomenology, that is, their attitudes, values and beliefs, is also crucial in deciding about the type of treatment sought and the extent to which people would comply with the curative regime. According to the Health Belief Model propounded by Rosenstock (1966, 1974), knowledge of patient's health-related beliefs is crucial for understanding the patient's psychological state of readiness to take specific action. For example, patients' compliance can be predicted considering their beliefs about severity, susceptibility and consequences of an illness, as well as the cost of a regimen and its likelihood of success (Becker & Maiman, 1975). Rosenstock originally proposed his health belief model to predict preventive health behaviour which was later on extended by Stretcher and Rosenstock (1997) to explain sick role behaviour as well.

Rosenstock's health belief model has primarily focused on beliefs which people have as individuals and ignored cultural beliefs which shape a person's beliefs about health and illness. There are important cultural beliefs (not incorporated in the health beliefs model) which have implications for understanding people's reaction to their sickness and subsequent coping, which are cultural beliefs about the causes of an illness. In the eastern cultures, people subscribe to many metaphysical beliefs as causes of their illness and as important factors in their recovery (Dalal, 1988, 2001, 2015). Cultural beliefs shape people's own theories about the causes of illness include, stress, some virus, physical imbalance, evil spirit, God's will and so on. These causal attributions tell us whether the patients will blame themselves, another person, situational factors or cosmic factors for the problem. For example, if a patient attributes his disease to some evil spirit, he would visit a priest, *ojha, pir* or some witch-doctor for the treatment. Contrarily, if patients attribute their illness to their own-selves (wrong habits or carelessness), they may feel guilt, may try to change their own behaviour and would show greater compliance to the treatment regimen (Dalal, 2006).

The psychomedical approach does not consider a patient as a passive recipient of the treatment but views him or her as an equal partner in the fight against the physical illness. Any treatment involves both the practitioner and the patient, and both need to cooperate in the complex venture. In the case of chronic disease, for example, the experience and knowledge of the patient may be of great value to the practitioners in deciding the future course of action. An ideal patient–practitioner relationship can dramatically enhance the efficacy of treatment and the process of a patient's recovery (Taylor, 2006). Patients, who are taught to be optimistic and are in control of their lives, get well quickly more completely than the passive and helpless ones. The new approach should transform rigid impersonal medical treatment to a more human, considerate one, where the patient is a partner in search for a cure. Cousins (1979) discovered that a sick person's most desperate need is contact on a personal level with his doctor, and an assurance that things are going to be alright.

An important distinction in the psychomedical approach is made between curing and healing. Curing is the removal of the disease, whereas healing implies psychological recovery of patients from some trauma. The emphasis in curing is on restoring the physical functioning of the body, healing on the other hand, focuses on restoring the psychological health of the patient by bringing changes in beliefs and expectations. A cancer patient might have been medically cured but his anxiety and sense of helplessness may persist for long, at times needing institutional help. In traditional Indian medical system, the distinction between curing and healing is clearly maintained. Even ordinary people maintain this distinction (Joshi, 1988; Kakar, 1982). Joshi, in his study in Central Himalayas, discovered that people make a distinction between *bis*, a primary, supernatural and actual cause and *bimari*, a secondary effect for which one gets medical treatment. Thus, when they go to a medical doctor, they talk about their physical condition and about physical symptoms which the doctor can cure. But when the same person goes to a priest, hakim, pir, ojha or vaidyas, he or she follows a different line. They talk more about emotional and psychic disorders to remove primary, supernatural and 'actual' causes of the disease. Thus, when a person falls sick, the measures for curing and healing are initiated simultaneously. In Indonesia, particularly in Bali, it is one of the responsibilities of a traditional healer to refer a patient to a medical doctor. Consequently, even when cured of the physical ailment, patients go to healers for holy water (Sinha, 1990). India, too, has a very rich tradition of healing practices (see Hasan, 1967; Kakar, 1982). Ayurvedic practitioners do combine healing and curing components of the treatment. The purpose of this chapter is not to discuss them at length, but to drive home a point that the psychomedical model has the potential to take care of both the healing and curing aspects of the treatment by attending to psychological and physical health, respectively. This provides enough scope to incorporate various features of our traditional health care system in the existing health programmes.

The psychomedical model envisions the possibility of involving social scientists, counsellors, spiritual leaders and traditional health practitioners in planning health care services. Public health is too serious a matter to be left only in the hands of medical professionals, who have no formal training in handling socio-cultural and psychological aspects of the illness. The health care system needs to be made broad based so that it can handle all the facets of the problem, including public education about health and hygiene. Apart from providing curative services, rural health centres should have been the nucleus of all round development. To achieve this dream, it is important that social workers, school teachers, religious leaders and even faith healers are closely associated with the activities of the health centres. Indonesian health services have shown the way, where traditional healers are trained to refer serious cases to medical professionals but these patients come back to the traditional healer for holy water, once they are cured. This system, thus, not only relieves pressure on the medical practitioners, but also takes care of both curing and healing aspects of the disease. Such a system may succeed in Indian conditions. The government statistics show that India has 5 million traditional practitioners which include vaidyas, homeopaths, Unāni and other folk health practitioners. These enormous resources have not been systematically utilized by the health planners so far.

One of the offshoots of the psychomedical model is the concept of self-healing which has not been given enough attention in health programmes. Everyone possesses self-curing and self-healing mechanism which is not properly recognized by the medical practitioners. In fact, medical science rarely pays attention to those who do not get sick or those who show remarkable recovery, defying all medical predictions. As many empirical studies show, the traditional health practices play a very important role in activating self-healing mechanism of the body by inducing proper psychological state (Anand, 2006, 2011). About 80 per cent of the illnesses are of self-limiting nature (WHO, 2011), well with the range of body's own healing powers. Thus, someone with the basic understanding of human mind can play a major role in alleviating a patient's suffering and in lessening the burden of medical professionals who can concentrate on serious illnesses. Para-professionals, yoga teachers and counsellors can provide good services to this end.

The psychomedical model is of much relevance in organizing community health services. A large number of community health programmes have failed in the past because they did not take into consideration local culture, community resources and expectations of the people. A careful understanding of the local community is necessary to mobilize their support and active involvement in health programmes. Early detection, secondary prevention and rehabilitation are the activities which local community can itself take over with minimum training, lessening their dependence on medical services. Such programmes will not only be cost-effective but also easily accessible and acceptable to those who would otherwise go unattended.

Promoting Health and Well-being

Asian systems focus on the advanced stages of development and states of well-being, and the Western systems provide the details of psychopathology and early development (see Leslie, 1998). Integrating these two perspectives may enable us with a 'full spectrum' model of health which traces aetiology, causes and treatment of illness (recovery) to maintain good health through various stages of growth and enlightenment.

The growth model focuses on the realization of the human potential for transcendent experiences and cultivation of wisdom that touches the higher levels of consciousness. In some way, the person works at the transpersonal level by recognizing continuity and interconnectedness of the living beings. The emphasis here is on higher order needs of the extended or inclusive self which are more encompassing. The pain and suffering of such a person have no bounds as they are not personal. Such kind of enlightenment seeks the common ground and gazes at the issues for all beings (*prāni*) and for everyone (*sarva*). Sharing and expanding the sense of self demands not only creativity but also discipline of a very high order. The journey from fragmentation to integration or from self to Self is very challenging but certainly capable of bringing unparallel joy and bliss. The vision celebrates the idea that "I am everywhere and everyone is in me." The differentiation is crossed in favour of integration. The person becomes more inward-looking, keen about transcending the vagaries of the physical environment and bodily (physical) concerns and focusing more and more on self-growth. Wellness then becomes a virtue (Conrad, 1994). In fact, this aspect of health is a major contribution of Indian positive psychology.

Normally, people are engaged in diverse social interactions and respond according to the specific demands. Their self-experience is often fragmented. The same person when engages in growth processes organizes his or her self and tries to rediscover the hidden potential. The person is empowered by recognizing his abilities to think, act and feel in an integrated fashion. It often occurs while one encounters a guru or gets guidance from some elder or by reading books or by engaging with relevant discourses. The company of noble people (*satsangati*) who are enlightened also contribute to well-being and growth.

Growth also involves vitality, thriving and a positive attitude. The recent developments in positive psychology clearly indicate that positive moods and feelings are not merely indicators of health, rather they contribute to it. They build and broaden the base for health. In other words, a person's happy or good mood not only exhibits his present health status but also leads to more happiness and positive health (Fredrickson, 2001). Increasingly, many studies show the effects of optimism and hope towards a person's well-being and health. Bonanno (2004) has shown in his work on resilience that we underestimate human capacity to thrive in very adverse life conditions. Unfortunately, the focus of research has largely been preoccupied with the negative aspects (illness and pathology) and the absence of disease has been treated as health. The studies on health, therefore, frequently use the measures that include the list of disorders and problems rather than positive aspects of health. It is in the case of quality of life and subjective well-being that attention is paid to the positive health.

Developments in positive psychology indicate that a growth orientation requires a change in the lifestyle, with a space for activities like meditation, yoga and looking within (Saligman, 2008). In today's stressful and tension-ridden life, these efforts contribute to peace, happiness and well-being of the people. The self of contemporary man is saturated with too much information and opportunities (Gergen, 1988, 1994). The market and media complicate the situation by drawing attention to the apparent achievements and attractions that disturb the equilibrium. It is, therefore, important to bring self-regulation and self-control in a relational world to the centre stage.

It is under the positive psychology movement that attention is now being paid to empathy, love, wisdom, gratitude, resilience and authenticity as aspects of well-being (see Snyder & Lopez, 2002). Viewing well-being in terms of pleasure or happiness is just one perspective.

There is another perspective that emphasizes on the actualization of human potential or one's true nature. The former presents the 'hedonic' view while the latter reflects 'eudaimonic' view (Ryan & Deci, 2001). The relationship of personal wellness and collective well-being is one area which needs serious attention. The social well-being as a positive state associated with optimal functioning within one's social network and community (Keyes, 1988) incorporates social integration, social contribution, social coherence, social actualization and social acceptance. The recent publications in this field (i.e., Diener & Biswas-Diener, 2008) have emphasized spiritual aspects of happiness and well-being.

These developments in the Western psychology have opened up the possibilities of integrating Indian and Western research to promote health and well-being of people globally. Traditional Indian health care systems which include both medicinal (Ayurvedic, herbal and so on) and folk-healing systems have thrived on human capacities to recover from the illnesses and emphasize on promoting positive human attributes. The Upanishads and other scriptures deal with the possibilities of the highest state of human existence and have discussed the methods of attaining it. If this knowledge could be assimilated with major discoveries and advances in the field of medicine, surgery and psychology in recent times, it would be a quantum jump forward, improving the quality of human existence. There are many exciting possibilities for research in this field.

2

History of Health and Healing Systems in India*

Health and healing have always been major concerns in the Indian civilization. The relics found from the excavation of ancient cities of Mohenjo-dāro and Harappa (now in Pakistan) reveal that the inhabitants were much concerned about maintaining good personal and public hygiene and were familiar with many medicinal plants to heal people from illnesses. In the later period, when Aryans settled in the north-west India, they not only started developing their own health and healing practices but also learnt a good deal from the natives also. Ayurveda was a well-formulated system of medicine by 5–6 century BCE, by the time of Gautam Buddha. Surgery was also widely practised by that time, as its textbook, the *Sushruta Samhitā*, evinces. Healing practices focused on both physical and mental health, which together in a holistic sense constitute well-being of an individual and also that of the society. The Vedas and Upanishads have extensively dealt with the ways to achieve an ideal state of health and well-being.

The *Sankhya* philosophy posits that it is the balance of three *gunas* (life attributes) within the individual which is important for maintaining the ideal level of well-being. Every person is believed to be constituted of three gunas called the *sattva* (purity and illumination), *rajas* (activity and affectivity) and *tamas* (passivity and darkness). These three gunas are associated with different physical and personality characteristics

---

* This chapter was written in collaboration with Jyoti Anand.

and, taken together, they determine temperament and physical constitution of a person. It is on the basis of the preponderance of one or the other gunas that people vary in terms of intelligence, activity or indolence, and thus experience different levels of well-being. It is the state of *sāmyavastha* or balance of three gunas that holds the secret of an individual's health and well-being (see Sinha, 1990).

According to the WHO (1978), health is a state of complete physical, mental and social well-being and is not merely the absence of a disease or infirmity. This definition of health is close to the way health is understood in ancient Indian medical texts. Sushruta, the ancient Indian surgeon, defined health as *prasannan-mendriyamanah swastha*. That is, health is a state of happiness and a feeling of spiritual, physical and mental well-being (Sharma, 1981, pp. 239–240). This health and well-being of an individual is conceived to be dependent on the well-being of all other creatures on the earth. An individual cannot be happy and healthy if there is suffering around him. This notion of interdependence is well illustrated in the invocation from the *Brihadāranyaka Upanishada* (1.4.14), which prays for the well-being of all living beings on earth. It goes like this, *Sarvey bhavantu sukhinah sarve santu nirāmayah, Sarve bhādrani pāshyantu mā kash-chid dukhābhag bhavet* (May all be happy; May all enjoy health and freedom from disease; May all have prosperity and good fortune; May none suffer or fall in evil days).

Charaka Samhitā, the ancient text on the Indian system of medicine, has designated the characteristics of happy (*sukhswarup*) and unhappy (*dukhswarup*) life. Life is said to be happy if the person is not afflicted with any somatic and psychic disorder, when the person is youthful, capable with strength, energy, reputation, manliness and prowess, possessing knowledge, specific knowledge and has efficient sense organs, having wealth and various favourable enjoyments, has achieved desired outcomes of all actions and moves about where he likes; contrary to it is unhappy life (30.22; also see Srivastava & Misra, 2011).

The popular term for health in Hindi language is 'swasthya', made up of two Sanskrit terms, *swa* (self) and *stha* (rooted, stationed)— implying 'one who is located in one's own self'. Health is thus, not only considered to be an internal state but also takes into consideration one's whole existence.

On the contrary, in spite of the wide popularity of the term 'healing', it has no equivalent in the Sanskrit language. There are terms such as happiness (*sukha*), fulfilment (*samridhi*), satisfaction (*santosh*), peace (*shānti*), health (swasthya), not-ill (*niroga*) and so on, but none of these terms encapsulates the essential meaning of the term 'healing'. The word 'healing' has its roots in the Latin word '*healan*', which connotes both the body and the spiritual element of the human being, as the things of healed. The Chambers Dictionary defines healing as 'becoming whole and healthy'. The Oxford English Dictionary defines it as 'to save, purify, cleanse, repair, mend'.

Thus, the term 'healing' may be understood in a broader sense as the *experience of an inner sense of well-being, harmony, balance and peace.* It is a process through which the harmony among mind, body and spirit is restored. It is in this sense that the terms 'swasthya' and 'healing' have many similar defining characteristics. Both entail reconstruction of the self, a change in attitude and (broadening of) one's vision and perspective. Thus, healing may not change the situation, but enables the individual to deal effectively with the crisis situation emanating from physical, supernatural and environmental conditions. Both 'swasthya' and 'healing' engender hope, acceptance, release of trapped psychic energy, resolution of internal conflicts and new insights.

The term 'healing' means more than recovery from illness; more than alleviation of physical pain. It also refers to relief from stress, anxiety, fear, guilt, loneliness and depression. Healing is a holistic term which implies a state of psycho-physical-spiritual well-being. Unlike modern medicine, healing primarily focuses on the people who suffer, not on the problem they suffer from. The scientific community and modern medicine are often critical and sceptical of the efficacy of such healing practices. Science rejects the supernatural. Folk healers are often alleged to be quacks, cheats who engage in dubious activities. Consequently, belief in such practices is attributed to ignorance, illiteracy and superstition. Despite all these aspersions, there is a proliferation of healing practices which cover the whole range of options—from alternative medicine to yoga therapy to faith healing.

Healing Practices in Pre-Vedic and Vedic Periods

As mentioned in the beginning, the earliest evidence of healing practices in India is from the relics and artefacts found from the cities of Harappa and Mohenjo-dāro. Harappan, or the Indus Valley Civilization as it is called, prospered on the banks of the Indus River and its tributaries in the western part of undivided India. It was a highly developed, stable and urban civilization which flourished for about 500 years, before the Aryans started settling in north India.

The healing practices of the Harappan civilization were compatible with the culture, beliefs and social practices of that time. The Harappans were animistic, as was evident from the artefacts of wild and tamed animals being worshipped, prominent among them was the bull. Emphasis on hygiene and ritualistic purity was evident from a bath and a toilet in almost every house, and from the presence of public baths. It was evident that shamans were part of the larger urban community, providing treatment for various diseases. As Zysk (1998) and Chattopadhyay (1982) noted, the healing paradigm of that period was that of magico-religious nature, in which evil spirits and rituals played an important role. Such ritualistic healing was performed through dancing, chanting, oblation, animal sacrifice and amulets, including administering local herbs. Various relics excavated from these twin cities of Harappa and Mohenjo-dāro reveal that the Mother Goddess (probably the earth) was worshipped to ward off bodily and natural calamities. A male God in a yoga posture, depicted with three faces and two horns, was also found in the excavation which very much resembles Shiva.

There are various theories about how such a well-developed urban civilization collapsed without leaving any traces of its existence until the excavation work started in the 1920s at the actual locations. There is no supportive evidence for the theory that Harappan civilization still existed when Aryan started migrating to the Indian subcontinent and got into conflict with the local inhabitants. It is quite likely that between 1900 and 1500 BCE, the Harappan civilization had gradually faded away when the Aryan culture was spreading throughout north India. In any case, the medico-religious model of healing continued to be the dominant ethos in the pre-and early-Vedic period. The Aryans who are believed to have migrated to India from Asia-minor, through Iran and Afghanistan, took another 2–3 centuries to settle in the northern India. As new settlers, they not only preserved and practised the medicinal knowledge they had accumulated during their migration but also imbued the local knowledge of plants and herbs in their healing practices.

These medicine men or healers were known as *bhisaj* in the Vedic period. These were male professionals "whose special craft was mending of the sick by removal of the disease demons and repairing of the injured part of the body." A bhisaj, like a shaman, a medicine man, or a diviner, possessed knowledge of medicinal plants, could recite the appropriate incantations and could enter into trance states, during which he trembled and danced (Zysk, 1998, p. 16). These bhisaj, however, were not considered at par with the priestly community. According to the Rigveda, in terms of hierarchy, they fell between carpenters (*taksans*) and priests (Brahmins). Like an uneducated carpenter, a bhisaj repaired injured or broken body parts, and like a priest, he had the knowledge of healing charms, rituals and invocations. One of the reasons why these bhisaj were not considered at par with the priestly class was because they travelled to distant places and came in direct contact with diseased persons, and thus they did not have ritualistic purity. The priestly class, for the same reason, was not supposed to practice medicine.

Thus, though Asvin brothers, the Gods' physicians, were praised in the Rigveda, they were debarred initially from partaking of the sacred Soma (drink offered to Gods), because they were in contact with diseased and impure human beings. But when the Gods needed Asvins' services to replace the head of a sacrifice, the Gods agreed to give them their share of Soma. For this, these two physicians had to go through the purification rites with the chanting of the *Bahispavamana Stotra* (hymns). It became an essential ritual, in the later period, of purification of the priestly healers. However, in general, the Vedic healers continued to be debarred from the religious practices, for being impure for coming in contact with diseased people, as the *Satapath Brahman* confirms. This kind of ambivalence about the status of bhisaj was evident in the Rigveda (RV:x.97.6) which held bhisaj as the healer of a disease, one who is knowledgeable of healing herbs. In the same verse, a bhisaj is mentioned as a *vipra*, a member of the priestly class. They were, however, included in the priestly class only after purification rituals. In the Yajurveda period, this ambivalent attitude towards bhisaj continued. The Yajurveda specifically states that a Brahmin must not practice medicine because a physician is impure and unfit to participate in *yagnas*. It should be clear that the Brahmins were discouraged from the practice of medicine, not from the use of medicine. In fact, the students of the Vedas were expected to learn 'about medicines, along with other subjects'.

In the later period, Manu clearly mentioned in his treatise, the *Manusmriti*, that no Brahmin should ever earn his living by medicine, logic or poison therapy unless in abject poverty, as these kinds of practices were held non-Vedic. It was in the later period when the Atharvaveda was fully accepted as the fourth Veda that the study of medicine was put on par with other Vedic subjects. However, this process of fully integrating the Atharvaveda in the fold of the Vedas was slow and took about 500 years. Though healers and vaidyas were respected for their specialized knowledge and skills, it was only in the later period that they were accepted at par with the priestly class. The Atharvaveda gave impetus to the enhanced status of the healers and their later integration within the Brahminical fold. Charaka advised that should anyone ask you (a vaidya) which of the Vedas to refer to, the answer is the Atharvaveda, because it deals with the treatment of diseases.

The fact remains that being out of the Brahminical social structure for almost a millennium, these nomadic healers were on the periphery of the mainstream community life of the Aryans. The Atharvaveda mentioned them as *cāranvaidya* (roving physicians). Organized in different sects and groups, depending on their specialization, many of these healers roamed the countryside and to far off places to practice their art and to gain knowledge about medicinal plants and healing techniques. These healers learnt from practical experience and by exchanging data with other healers. That is the reason that they were also coming in contact with non-Aryans in their travels to learn about new plants, herbs and modes of treatment. These contacts with non-Aryans further bolstered the belief that they are impure. This was not palatable to the post-Vedic Brahminical orthodoxy, but in the later period, ways were found to consecrate and induct these cāranvaidya back in their fold.

Again, these roaming physicians frequently came in contact with the wandering ascetics called *śravanas*. These śravanas had abandoned the society to seek liberation from the endless cycles of birth and death and did not care for the ritualistic practices of brahminical class. The roaming physicians freely associated with these śravanas who were more favourably disposed towards healing art. The close association between these roaming physicians and Buddhist śravanas was more evident in the later period. Megasthenes, the Greek traveller who came to India in 300 BCE, depicted the ascetic physician as living away from the habitats, being frugal, practicing austerity and living on the offered food. This specification fits for both Ayurvedic practitioner and Buddhist monks living in *sanghas* (Buddhist monasteries).

Eventually, the Aryans moved eastward from Punjab to the north-west region, towards the Gangetic plains where they established small kingdoms with distinct socio-cultural and linguistic ethos. It was a period when diverse cultures were interacting in small kingdoms and urban centres and there was growing awareness of the influence of lifestyle, environment and supernatural on health and well-being. In such a context, in the region east of the confluence of Ganga and Yamuna, Buddhism, Jainism and other new ascetic and philosophical movements made waves. Many of these movements promoted the free spirit of enquiry and experimentation in all fields of knowledge, including the medicine. We find early Buddhist and Jaina texts in *Prakṛit* (also in Pali and other vernacular languages), describing the use of medicines, surgical procedures, trepanation, purges and emetics, practices, integrating them into the existing social order and value system. The early medical texts also recognized the importance of cultivating compassion and humanistic values as being essential for health and well-being.

The Buddha himself was seen as the 'healing guru' (*Bhaishajyaguru*) and healing practices were part of the Buddhist monastic tradition. Monastic infirmities were established to cater to both sick monks and lay persons. Buddhist monks disseminated Indian medical knowledge from Persia and Central Asia to China and South-east Asia. Buddhism also took with it medical knowledge to southern regions of the sub-continent, to Sri Lanka, especially during and after the reign of Ashoka, the Great. Chinese Buddhist traveller Fa-Hsien who came to India in the fifth century AD reported that in Patliputra trading class established many shelters and healing centres for poor, destitute and diseased. They were given food and care, were attended by vaidyas and were given medicine without any charge. There were *arogyashālās* (health centres) in the whole India, for which kings, rich and affluent, generously donated for nursing and treating sick people of all classes and communities. Taxila (now in Pakistan) and Nalanda Universities were the major centres for the study of Ayurveda and training of vaidyas by that time. Buddhist monasteries, temples and shrines had become the major nodal centres for practicing Ayurveda and attending to the sick. By the tenth century, medicinal practices were largely integrated with religious centres, both in Southern and Northern India.

Two Streams of Traditional Medicine

By the time of Buddha (600 BCE), the divide between two distinct healing systems was discernible. One was that of Ayurvedic and ascetic healing and the other one being that of folk tradition. These two ancient systems belong to different strata of the society, having different world views and ways of living and healing. Whereas Ayurveda became a formal system of Indian medicine, folk-healing practices remained an informal system with no known proponents or institutions to support.

The distinction made between great and small tradition by Marriot (1955) can be relevant in this context. The great tradition was primarily based on the Ayurvedic theories and practices and was supported by both the Brahminical and, later, by the Buddhist order. By the time of Buddha, Ayurveda was well established as a medical system of India and its popularity was rising. In fact, when Jivak was appointed as the physician of Buddha by King Bimbisara of Magadha (part of Bihar at that time), a big population of the city turned to Buddhism to be able to get treatment from him.

Contrarily, the folk-healing tradition was primarily subscribed by people who were out of the Brahminical fold, those who were from the lower strata, mountain and forest dwellers, naked (uncivilized) and the like. The medical knowledge of such primitive healers was considered to be that of magico-religious nature and was, in a way, the continuation of the practices of non-Aryans. Based on animal sacrifice, obscure rituals, malevolent and benevolent spirits, emulates, herbs and other social rites, these primitive practices were seen with scepticism and were shunned by the Brahminical class. At the initial stages of its development, Ayurveda derived a good deal from this informal folk knowledge source. In due course, many of the non-Aryan practices were learnt by the wandering healers and were later adopted by the post-Vedic medical practitioners. However, in adapting these non-Aryan practices within the Brahminical fold, these healing practices went through a metamorphosis. They became a part of the ritualistic procedure involving the invocation of higher deities, chanting and elaborate healing procedure while administrating the medicine. Charaka writes in the *Charaka Samhitā* that on the completion of his studies, a physician is called 'twice born' (like Brahmins) and acquires the title of Vaidya.

Ayurvedic theories and practices mark a paradigm shift in healing practices in India. With the development of Ayurveda, the medical paradigm shifted from the magico-religious to logico-empirical approach. As Zysk (1998) stated, this transition was possible because of the close association between the wandering medicine men and heterodox ascetics. These medicine men were moving in the countryside, administering the cure to all those who required, closely watching the effect of medication and exchanging valuable information with other fellow healers. The wandering ascetics (śravanas) were also searching for explanations of nature and life in their own ways. As they were out of the Brahminical fold, they had more freedom to base their medicinal knowledge on direct observations or learning from folk practitioners. Chattopadhyay (1982) argues that such empirical, data-based rational analysis led to the development of sound medical epistemology that is unique to Indian medicine. Their empirical orientation also led to the inclusion of environmental factors, daily routine and social factors in their understanding of causality and remedy of the diseases (Zysk, 1998).

As during their wide travelling, these wandering vaidyas continued to be in contact with local healers, an ambivalent attitude towards them continued. Local healers were a major source of information and learning for these vaidyas. Knowledge about new diseases and medicinal herbs was important for them. This closed contact between these two classes of healers was not approved by the priestly class. Manu wrote in the *Manusmriti* (in the first century BCE) very strongly that it is bad to eat food offered, even as alms by a medicine man or a surgeon, for it is like taking food from polluted people, such as hunters, whores, bird-catchers and eunuchs. Manu also ruled that food offered by a surgeon is as filthy as offered by a blacksmith. This could be because Susrut advised surgeons to get their instruments made of good iron by a blacksmith. The *Maitri Upanishad* branded the practitioners of poison treatment as heretics, unfit for higher status. Such expertise was probably more prevalent among the healer of the lowest strata of the society.

Clearly, by the time of Buddha (sixth and fifth century BCE), cleavages widened between bhisaj or vaidya who were practicing Ayurveda and folk healers. These folk healers were mostly non-Aryans, living in forests and remote areas, or were those engaged in menial work. Because they were living closer to the nature, they were efficient in the treatment of natural calamities, such as treatment of poisoning and snake-biting, bone-fixing, wound healing and so on. They were more frequently engaged in sorcery, spirit-possession and other magico-religious practices.

These two systems of healing fell further apart in the later period when Ayurveda got fully integrated within the Brahminical fold. Ayurveda accepted the authority of the Vedas, particularly that of the Atharvaveda, and its accompanying magico-religious and ritualistic practices. Many scholars argue that this was merely a superimposition in the later period on the scientific-empirical ethos of Ayurveda (Kakar, 1982; Misra, 2004; Svoboda, 1992).

Chattopadhyaya (1982), in his commentary on the *Charaka Samhitā*, writes that metaphysics and supernatural contents introduced in it, including those of karma and unseen causes, are loosely superimposed on its otherwise scientific content. By the beginning of the post-AD period, the study of Ayurveda was considered to be at par with that of the Vedas. The *Charaka Samhitā* and the *Sushruta Samhitā* were accepted as standard texts of the Indian system of medicine. This official patronage and acceptance by the Brahminical class led to the unhindered growth of the Indian system of medicine and surgery in the later period. Buddhist influence can be seen on classic text on Ayurveda, the *Ashtangahrdayam* composed by the Buddhist monk Vagbhata.

The healing practices and medicine men of the lower stratum of the society rarely had this kind of patronage. These folk practices, however, continued to survive and grow in a natural process and on the basis of popular support. Such folk practices range from home remedies related to nutrition and treatment for minor ailments to more sophisticated procedures such as midwifery, bone setting and physical and mental disorders. Folk knowledge of healing was preserved through folklores and mythology. It was transmitted from one generation to another in the absence of any documentation. Many of such skills and expertise were needed by all sections of the society, as evident in various episodes of the *Mahābhārat* and Puranic texts. It is quite likely that much of this folk knowledge of medicine was lost in the long history and was hardly ever documented in the past.

It might be noted that though these two systems of healing practices were distinct, there was no open rivalry; an undercurrent of suspicion and competition was always there. From the Vedic time, there was substantial cross-fertilization, mutual leaning and acceptance. The folk healers served to that section of the society which did not have access to professionally trained vaidyas and surgeons. Both the

Charaka Samhitā and the *Sushruta Samhitā* urge physicians to seek the help of cowherds, hunters and forest-dwellers for procuring and preparing medicinal plants.

One thing which was common between Ayurveda and folk practices was that both the systems discouraged practicing medicine for livelihood. The *Charaka Samhitā* does not approve professionalization of medical practice, meaning thereby, it should not be used for earning a livelihood. The *Charaka Samhitā* mentions that those who practice medicine out of compassion, not for gains and gratification, stand above all others. Those for the sake of making a living trade in medicine are bargaining for the dust heap, forsaking a heap of gold (*Charaka Samhitā*). Patients are also advised not to be led by the exaggerated claims of quacks, who were not properly trained vaidyas.

Emergence of the Ayurveda

Ayurveda has no known beginning as a system of medicine. The early Vedic approach of attributing diseases to evil spirits and engaging in unexplainable rituals, recitations from the Vedas, charms use of some medicinal plants to a sophisticated, scientific medical system with specialized textbooks was a long journey for the Ayurveda. It was a journey which was three millennia-long with many ups and downs.

There are three different mythological stories about the origin of Ayurveda in the Indian scriptures. First is *Brahma*, the creator of the universe, who passed on this knowledge to *Prajapatis* (who manage different parts of the universe), from whom the Aswins learnt and further taught it to Indra. Later, Indra passed it on to Rishi Bharadwaj to heal the sick on earth. Second is the mythology of *Samundra Manthana* (Churning of the Ocean), as described in the *Puranas* and the *Mahābhārata*. Both, demons and Gods, decided to churn the Kshira Sagar (Ocean of Milk) to find nectar. Many divine objects and beings emerged from the Ocean as the churning continued; the last to emerge was Dhavantary with a pitcher of nectar. Dhanvantary is considered to be the avatar of Lord Vishnu. Dhanvantary is held as the most ancient God of Ayurveda, who holds Ayurvedic inscriptions in one hand and some herbs in the other. All vaidyas in India worship him on the day of Dhanateras, which falls two days before the Deepawali festival.

The third story goes like this. Many sages, at one point of time, got seriously concerned about the diseases and disorders from which the humanity was suffering and wanted to find ways to heal. They decided to hold a medical conference, somewhere in the Himalayan region, inviting sages and medicine men from all over. Sage Bharadwaj took the initiative to hold this international conference. The names of sages who participated in this conference are listed in *Charak Samhitā* (1.1 8–14). They discussed for days about the herbs and plants having medicinal values, and also about other ways to deal with health problems. They also decided at the end of the conference to send Sage Bharadwaj as there representative to Indra, who was considered the most knowledgeable about the science of healing. Sage Bharadwaj learnt it from Indra and, in turn, taught this science to Atrey and others (see Raina, 1990). This story seems to be just a variant of the first one.

Many scholars of Ayurveda have argued that these mythological stories about the origin of Ayurveda mentioned in the Puranas and other texts are later constructions, superimposed on the scientific body of medicinal knowledge. This cosmology of Ayurveda, as included in the *Charaka Samhitā*, starkly stands out and, otherwise, incompatible with the empirical approach of Ayurveda. Nevertheless, it served the purpose of assimilating Ayurveda within the Brahminical fold, and this process continued for almost a millennium.

Ayurveda, in reality, had no known fixed beginning, and as stated earlier, grew in the natural course with time. The Rigveda and the Atharvaveda have referred to some foundational features of Ayurveda. According to the Rigveda, diseases mainly occur due to the imbalance of the three bodily attributes, called '*tri-dhatu*', also known as '*tridosas*'. These are *vāta* (wind), *pitta* (body acids) and *kapha* (phlegm). However, the Atharvaveda states the same 'tridosa-theory' in a somewhat different manner. According to the Atharvaveda, diseases are caused by three elements, namely, *abhraja* occurring due to moisture-ladden cloud which indicates the excess of kapha element, *vataja* happening due to wind and *susmaja* indicating pitta or fiery element in the body. The Atharvaveda also discusses the four types of *chikitsā* (treatment). The *Atharvāna Chikitsā* deals with the chanting of mantras. It is known as faith healing by way of psychiatry or psychotherapy or psychological type of treatment. The *Angirāsa Chikitsā* mainly discusses about the medical treatment based on the application of medicinal herbs and products of animals and birds. *Daivi Chikitsā* states about curing diseases with the help of natural elements such as sunrays, water, earth and so on. *Ausadhi Chikitsā* is the treatment by medicines. The Atharvaveda, thus, deals with the human anatomy, classification of diseases, herbal medicines and its application.

As the scriptures show, Ayurveda was first compiled as a text by Agnivesha, in his work the *Agnivesh Tantra* in the Vedic times. He was one of the pupils of Rishi Atreya who was taught Ayurveda by Rishi Bharadwaj. Many scholars in the later period kept on adding to this original treatise and the *Charaka Samhitā* may be a compilation of this medicinal knowledge. Chattopadhyaya (1982) is of the views that the *Charaka Samhitā*, in its original form, is not the work of one person but is a compilation of medical knowledge of the roving physicians. The Samhitā itself refers to different approaches to medicine and describes numerous medical traditions. The word 'Charaka' means a wanderer, with Sanskrit root 'car' (to wander), an apt referral to ascetic sramans and roving medicine men. The fifth-century Chinese work *Sūtrālamkāra* mentions Charaka as a physician of King Kanishk of Kushan Dynasty who ruled in north-west India in the first century AD. It is quite possible that Charaka might have been a roaming-sraman in King Kanishk's court who may have participated in editing and compiling an already existing body of medical knowledge. Whatever the case may be, the precise timing of the compilation of the *Charaka Samhitā* is not known. The available evidence suggests that it existed in the first century AD, along with *Sushruta Samhitā*, *Ashtāngahrdayam*, *Ashtāngasamgraha*, *Bhela Samhitā* and *Kashyapa Samhitā*. A large number of texts and commentaries were added in the later period.

Ayurveda has survived a long history of three millennia and is still widely practised in India. One of the major reasons for the continued practice of Ayurveda has been that it has always remained a living tradition which was never resistant to change. As Svoboda (1992, p. 21) writes, "Over the centuries mainstream Ayurvedic beliefs and practices have deviated substantially from those of the ancient texts." Because of this flexibility, there have been many schools and systems in Ayurveda, though only a few have survived in the present times. As an individualized science, each practising vaidya within the Ayurvedic system has enough flexibility to tailor-make the therapy for each patient, keeping in view a holistic assessment of the patient and of her/his personality and needs.

Ayurvedic Theory of Well-being

It is believed that the Ayurveda, as communicated by Brahma to Prajapati consisted of 100,000 verses into 1,000 chapters, which Sage Bharadwaj brought to the earth for humanity. No one can verify the veracity of this belief. As we know, the Atharveds has a large number of verses, out of which about 114 verses form the basis for the beginning of Ayurveda. As mentioned earlier, this growing body of medicinal knowledge was compiled in the *Charaka Samhitā*. According to the *Charaka Samhitā*, the original text was lost and was restored later by a Kashmiri Drdhabala, who added 17 chapters to the sixth section, as well whole of the eighth section. In this new addition, many of the disconnected materials were brought together and revised (Zimmer, 1951). In the present version of the *Charaka Samhitā*, there are eight sections, having 120 chapters. These sections (*Sthāna*) are: (a) Sutra Sthāna (general principles), (b) Nidhan Sthāna (pathology, causes), (c) Viman Sthāna (diagnostics), (d) Sharir Sthāna (anatomy, metaphysics), (e) Indriya Sthāna (prognosis), (f) Chikista Sthāna (treatment), (g) Kalp Sthāna (pharmacy) and (h) Siddhi Sthāna (purification and growth).

Ayurveda is the principal architect of the Indian concepts of the person and the body. For Ayurveda, spirit and matter, soul and body, although different, are not alien, insofar as they can be brought together in a healthy relationship with consequences that are mutually beneficial. Its prime concern is not with 'healing' in the narrow sense of curing illness but in the broader sense of promoting health, well-being and longevity. According to Kakar (2003), the emphasis on the wholeness of the person is reflected in the comprehensiveness of the diagnostic examination. An Ayurvedic practitioner not only checks up for pathological conditions and demography but also checks up for vitality, digestive power, emotional and mental state, personality and family condition.

According to the *Charaka Samhitā*, a person is a microcosm of the cosmos; all that are in the person are also present in the universe, and vice versa. The cosmos is believed to be constituted of six elements—earth, fire, wind, water, ether and Brahman. These elements also constitute the person. Because these elements are present in different proportions in each person, each one has a different temperament. Thus, each person needs a different treatment plan for healing.

In Ayurveda, any disturbance, physical or mental, manifests itself both in the somatic and in the psychic spheres, through the intermediary process of the vitiation of the 'humours'. Ayurvedic therapy aims at correcting the doshas or the imbalances and derangements of the bodily humours (namely, vāta or bodily air, pitta or bile, and kapha or phlegm) and restoring equilibrium. It does so by coordinating all of the material, mental and spiritual resources of the whole person, recognizing that the essence of these potencies is manifestation of cosmic forces. Medical intervention at the physical level is of four types: diet, activity, purification and palliation (Svoboda, 1992). In essence, the maintenance of equilibrium is health and, conversely, the disturbance of the equilibrium of tissue elements characterizes the state of the disease.

While treating patients, Ayurvedic physician conducts two types of examinations, first that of the patient (*rogi parikshā*) and second that of the disease (*roga parikshā*). The patient is examined in totality, checkup of the bodily state (location of disease, issues, digestion, metabolism, pulse, urine, faeces, tongue, eyesight and so on), constitution (age, dietary habits and so on), living place, surrounding, heredity, climate and season. The disease is examined in terms of deficiency or excess, nutrition, nature and symptoms, pain and other discomforts. Ayurvedic physicians knew that the disease can also be caused by small organisms, called *kirmi*, in the Ayurvedic texts. These kirmis could be visible, like insects, flies, worms or may be invisible, about which inferences can be drawn by watching patient's condition and symptoms. Sushruta mentioned how infectious diseases are spread by a variety of means, including inhalation, ingestion, sexual intercourse and body contact. There was no microscope those days and there were no ways of knowing the exact nature of the invisible creatures.

After a comprehensive examination of the person and disease, the treatment was prescribed, which included avoidance of causative factors, medicine, regulated diet, activities and other precautions. According to Ayurveda, good health is dependent on daily activities (*achar*), leisure and relaxation (*vihar*), nutritional diet (*ahar*) and right thoughts and attitudes (*vichar*). To maintain good health, one should become aware of own body, emotion and thoughts, cultivate proper dietary habits, make breathing quiet and deep, and calm down one's own mind and focus it inwardly. The Ayurvedic model of well-being shows how body, mind and spirit interactions can be predicted, balanced and improved to enable us to live happily and harmoniously.

Ayurvedic medicinal knowledge is quite extensive. There are numerous evidences that extensive and in-depth studies are being done on a plant before that was included into the body of medical knowledge. Sometimes such testing continued even for many decades or centuries before medicinal formulation was authenticated by the experts. This process included aspects like classification and nomenclature of root plants and herbs, methods of purification, contraindications, the effect on physiological systems, the effect on body tissues, the effect on organs, the effect on the excretory system, qualities, metabolic activity, post-digestive effect, drug therapeutic class and administrating schemes. Different sections of Ayurveda clearly spell out these aspects. There are around 25,000 plant drug formulations in the codified Ayurvedic system.

Folk Tradition of Healing

Folk tradition refers to a set of beliefs, attitudes and actions shared by a cultural group, which also determine world views and relationships (Thomas, 2001). It explains how a community attempts to develop ecologically valid understanding of human nature; human suffering and remedial measures (Kleinman, 1988). In many anthropological texts (e.g., Mariott, 1955), folk practices are considered within the little tradition, that is, the beliefs and practices of the masses. Shamans, spirits and local deities are all part of it.

The question as to 'what is folk healing' has no concise and categorical answer. In most of the cases, folk healing is understood, vis-à-vis, Western medicine, and this comparison forms the basis of understanding these two modes of healing practices. There are many alternative terms which are used to connote folk healing—indigenous, native, aboriginal, primitive, traditional, local and faith healing. Most of the ethnographic research in the colonial era considered these folk therapies as unscientific, esoteric, demonic, superstitious, placebos and similar labels (Simpson, 2001). They are looked upon with suspicion by urban, educated and scientific-minded population. The work of Kakar (1982, 2003) and Kleinman (1980, 1988) has shown that most of these traditional practices are deeply entrenched in folk wisdom and sound theories of mind. They provide practical solutions to personal, familial and social problems and have been integrated into the communal life.

A similar situation prevailed in India two millennia back when Ayurveda was fully established and practised as a rational-empirical system of medicine. Folk healing was viewed as primitive by the practitioners of Ayurveda. The *Mahābhārata* and the *Rāmāyana* mention about forest tribes, such as Koel, Bhil, Kirat, Kevat and also the serving class who were at the lower rung of the social hierarchy. Many of these tribes were pre-Aryans and had developed their own healing practices and rituals. These healing practices have no recorded history, no known proponents, no divine beginning, no text to follow and no official patronage. Their growth was always organic, based on trial and error, and personal experience. This knowledge was carried forward from one generation to another through inheritance or apprenticeship. This knowledge remained a part of the oral culture throughout the history and was preserved through folktales, folklores, myths and legends. The songs, dances, proverbs, ceremonies, sacred rituals, invocations and festivals remained vehicles to transmit folk knowledge over the centuries. Folk and Ayurvedic practices peacefully coexisted, though an undercurrent of mutual mistrust always remained. Of course, in the long history due to local influences, there are distortions, diversions and mutations in folk practices on the negative side, and improvisations, adaptations and innovations on the positive side (Dalal, 2011).

There is no denying the fact that there were abundant sources of medical know-how in the society, which accumulated since time immemorial. Some of them were later codified into the canonical texts of Ayurveda, but otherwise, they mostly remained fragmented, informal and region-specific. Since folk practitioners mostly came from the lower strata of the society, having no authority and power or scholarly aura, they remained distant from the Brahminical ethos. Yet, as many of the healers specialized in specific healing techniques, they were in demand and were respected. For example, it is not uncommon for experienced vaidyas to seek the help of folk healers in paediatric care, poison therapy or spirit possession. Classical Ayurveda has been enriched over centuries through such interactions and exchange with folk practitioners. Though these two systems were distinct and independent, there was no marked hostility or rivalry between the two in ancient India. In fact, there are more references of mutual respect and complementarity.

Folk healing comprises a large variety of remedies to deal with human suffering. These remedies ranged from home preparations for the nutritional deficiency to treating minor illnesses, to more sophisticated procedures, such as midwifery, bone setting and treatment of snake bites and mental disorders. There were also specialists in blood-letting, experts in physical medical practices and others with intimate knowledge of medicinal plants. Some healing practices were considered to be sacred and were associated with rituals that helped safeguard them. It is interesting to note that in folk systems, there is a considerable overlapping between healing plants and sacred plants, and certain healing plants were venerated. Rituals and supernatural were always of the folk practices and many such rituals were adopted from Ayurveda. The reverse was also true. Mahasweta Devi (2002) has convincingly argued that Kāli was a tribal Goddess who was co-opted by the upper class.

Traditional healers do not undertake medical service as a full-time vocation; the typical healer may be a farmer, a barber, a shopkeeper, a blacksmith or even a wandering monk. Its low sustenance cost is one of the reasons why the folk healing is so widespread across India and survived for so long. According to the patients, their belief in the good heart and genuine mind of the healer is essential for healing to be effective. Becoming a folk healer is not a conscious independent personal decision of the healer. It is a responsibility inherited or entrusted by the community. It is also an honour which has to be earned. Each culture and society determines their own healers based on the commitment, sacrifice, skills, abilities and inner goodness of the prospective healers. These healers must also be well versed in the ancient ways of their ancestors. Of course, there were cheats and quakes in both the systems who would make tall claims of their healing prowess. The *Charaka Simhitā* implores people to be cautious of such healers.

Characteristic Features of Indian Healing Systems

The separate healing systems, Ayurveda and folk healing share many common characteristics. These are termed as great and little traditions of healing, which have emerged and prospered within larger Indian cultural background and share a common history and concerns. Though these two healing systems have existed on their own, they have mutually enriched each other throughout the history. Both are now considered as an integral part of Indian systems of healing. Here, some of the common features of Ayurveda and folk healing are identified and discussed (for details, see Anand and Dalal [2013]).

1. **Embedded in the Larger Belief System:** Health beliefs in India seldom stand independent of the other indigenous beliefs. They, in many ways, are intricately weaved into the other community beliefs about child rearing, marriage, personal tragedies and morality. From the ontological standpoint, health is integral to the very fact of living and dying. Health from the Indian perspective is seen as part of the general well-being of the individual. It is also contended that individual well-being is also contingent on happiness and well-being of others in the family and social network and that of other living beings. Health is thus not considered to be an individual problem only but is also presumed to affect social life of the whole community.

2. **Cultural Compatibility:** It should be noted that indigenous systems generally combine medicinal treatment with cultural beliefs and social practices. The healing properties of many Ayurvedic medicines are well acknowledged in the pharmaceutical research and so is the remedial efficacy of many herbal prescriptions. What is worth noting is that these indigenous medicinal treatments are rooted in the faith and beliefs of the local communities. The plausible explanations for the ailments focus not only on the bodily conditions but also on the mental state of the patient and a shared belief system. Prevalent socio-spiritual beliefs, rituals and practices create the necessary conditions for fostering a positive mental state of hope, optimism and initiative. They serve as important inner resources to combat illness and other related adversities, and thereby enhance the efficacy of indigenous medicine (Kleinman, 1980).

3. **Holistic Approach:** Both healing systems are holistic in their approach. They aim at the overall well-being of the person. The focus of healing is the person, not on their problems per se. Healers know that mind, body and spirit are in a dynamic equilibrium and one part cannot remain healthy without the other. Holistic approach takes into consideration values, emotions, beliefs, social interaction and spiritual orientation of a person in their healing practices.

Most of the healers from both systems know from their personal experience that treating the person is not enough. Unless the family and the community to which the person belongs change, any improvement in his or her mental health will be short lived. Very often, the problems for which people come to a healer have their genesis in unhealthy social relationships. It is, therefore, imperative that all concerned parties participate in the healing process.

Indians have a propensity to believe in the metaphysical causation of the poor health, as is confirmed in many studies (Dalal, 2000a, 2015). It is thus generally believed that physical and mental health problem may be the outcome of economic, social and moral crises a person is undergoing, and that just medicinal treatment will not bring the person back to sound health status. People go to the same healer for their health problems, as well for other wide-ranging problems they face in personal life, including those of business loss or marital discord (Kakar, 1982). This holistic view of health is deeply embedded in the traditional belief system and health practices of the society.

4. **Restoring Equilibrium:** In both the healing systems, the implicit assumption is that men are embedded in the environment they live in. Therefore, a harmonious relation between man and environment is essential for healthy living. This inclusive view also recognizes the continuity of the body and universe. The continuity of microcosm and macrocosm and there sharing in terms of five basic elements (*pancha mahābhutas*) of which both are made. The interconnectedness and complementarity inherent in nature is the key to unlock the principles of health and well-being.

   Healing also entails restoring equilibrium between the mundane and supernatural worlds. Gods, ancestors and evil spirits are all considered be the part of the healing process, more in the case of folk healing than in Ayurveda. Different healing practices use different forms of sacred rituals (not religious) and certain rituals are part of the complete cure of the person.

5. **Healing as a Social Service:** Throughout the history, healing and curing remained as a service offered by the knowledgeable people. It was not considered as a profession, not as a means of livelihood. In fact, folk healers and vaidyas have some other work or occupation for their livelihood. Healing services offered to the needy were part of their social obligation, for which they were

not supposed to charge. They were often compensated in terms of offerings by the families and communities, once the person has healed. Ayurvedic scriptures proscribe changing for the healing services, as is mentioned in the earlier sections. This practice of not charging a fee for healing services is not unique to India but was prevalent in all traditional and aboriginal societies in other countries (Gielen, Fish & Draguns, 2004). In the market culture of the today's world, this scenario has starkly changed.

Medical Pluralism in India

Bhasin (2007) defined medical pluralism as

> the synchronic existence in a society of more than one medicine system grounded in different principles or based on different worldviews. Medical pluralism offers a variety of treatment options that health seekers choose to utilize exclusively, successively, or simultaneously.

In different regions of India, multiple therapy systems and diversity of health practices coexist. Apart from the folk and Ayurvedic systems of medicine, prominent ones which have a significant presence are Unāni, homeopathy, Siddha, naturopathy, Yoga, Tibetan and Siddha system of healing. In due course of history, these systems are integrated with Ayurveda and folk systems or coexisted as a distinct one. The government has created in recent years a separate department for some alternative system of medicine called AYUSH which comprises Ayurveda, Yoga, Unāni, Siddha and Homeopathy.

Among the alternative systems, except Unāni and homeopathy, all other systems are home-grown and converge with Ayurveda. The Unāni system of medicine is based on the teachings of Greek physicians Hippocrates and Galen, and in the later period, developed into an elaborate medical system as it moved to Arab countries and Iran in the middle age. It was popularly known as the Islamic medicinal system and was brought to India by the Muslim invaders in eleventh to twelfth centuries. The Unāni system thrived in India during the Delhi Sultanate and was later spread all over India during the Mughal Empire. The Unāni medicine is based on the concept of the four humours: phlegm (*balgham*), blood (*dam*), yellow bile (*safrā'*) and black bile (*saudā'*). Accurate pulse reading (*nādi parikshana*) is considered very important in the Unāni medicinal system. There were many eminent Unāni practitioners, known as hakims, in the long history. As a regular practice, many hakims include Ayurvedic medicines in their treatment of the patients.

Homeopathy was founded by a German doctor Samuel Hahnemann at the beginning of the nineteenth century. India is one country in which homeopathy received an amazing acceptance as an alternative system of medicine. A major advantage of homeopathic therapy is its simplicity of learning and the quick possibilities for self-help. The philosophical ideas of homeopathy are easy to grasp and then the less cost of treatment goes in its favour.

In India, the patients often choose the therapies according to their accessibility, affordability and personal preference. Moreover, the success story of the AYUSH therapies is explained by the support of the political administration, the financial satisfaction and active participation of the patients. But, mainly in rural areas, the choice of treatment depends on the availability according to time and distance as well as cost effectiveness. These alternate systems of medicine fit well in a pluralist culture of India with the immense diversity of diet, habits, social practices and belief systems.

Modern Medicine and Indigenous Systems

For the last three millennia, though, both Ayurveda and folk healing remained competing systems of health and well-being, they also complemented each other in rendering services to the masses in India. Because of their cultural compatibility and mass support, they continued to flourish till the modern period. As mentioned earlier, the medial plurality has been Indian ethos and many other different systems were accepted by the masses as an alternative mode of treatment. These alternate systems never posed any threat to the mass-base of Ayurveda and folk healing. But the case of Western medicine, which is also known as allopathy or modern medicine or scientific medicine, was different.

The modern scientific medicine has built on the advances in biological sciences and human physiology in the last two centuries (Capra, 1983). It is based on the Cartesian proposition that mind and body are separate, started focusing on body as a machine, ignoring psychological, social and environmental aspects of illness. This reductionist approach considers disease and injuries as a breakdown of the bodily mechanism. Disease is held as caused by the invasion of microbes, and thus the focus of treatment is on antibiotics and chemical-based medicines to deal with these microorganisms.

The modern medicine grew rapidly in the West in the nineteenth century with many scientific discoveries and growing knowledge about microorganisms. The period of rapid industrialization and urbanization in Europe, and along with that many epidemic diseases, like cholera, small-pox, tuberculosis and typhoid which resulted in mass mortality in the cities. It led to the development of public health care programmes and of the institutions of modern medicine (Porter, 2002). There were institutionalization and bureaucratization of medical service. Instead of patient's home, medical activities shifted to the doctor's office, hospital, medical colleges and laboratories. Medical treatment and practices standardized with a division of labour and role marking various services. Medicine gradually became a profession than a social service as it was known earlier.

The same medical model became a prototype when the West started colonizing other regions of the world. After the colonial rule, the East India Company initially and the British government later propagated Western medicine in India. They had no familiarity with the Indian medical practices and needed treatment facility for their army and administrators. The physicians and surgeons who came along with the colonial rulers did establish hospitals in their cantonments, the facilities which were extended to colonial local collaborators also. There were many tropical and other diseases for which services of indigenous practitioners were also sought. The Christian missionaries who arrived later on contributed to the spread of Western medicine in India. Keeping their primary objective of converting local population to Christianity, the missionaries concentrated more on rural and tribal regions (Gupta, 1998). They started clinics and hospitals for the local people. Missionaries engaged in a big way to start leprosy centres and lunatic asylums to get their entry into the community. The colonial government also established hospitals, mostly in their residencies for the local people, as the British rule expanded all over India. There was a need to control epidemic diseases, such as malaria, plague, typhoid and cholera. For example, plague epidemic killed more than two million in the last decade of the nineteenth century and there was a dire need to control its spread.

It is argued that the Indians accepted British law with comparative ease but not the British medicine (McRobert, 1929; Royle, 1837). The response was basically three-pronged: (a) conformism, (b) defiance and (c) quest for alternatives. Urban upper and middle class, which were in greater contact with the colonial government, patronized Western medicine, but for the larger population, indigenous treatment systems were cheap and accessible. The voice of 'defiance' slowly ended and became a voice on 'defence' of the indigenous system. At some level, the critique of Western medicine became a tool of protest against the colonial rule. In any case, in later years, it became difficult to ignore and oppose the Western medicine which was the dominant mode of treatment in government hospitals.

Notwithstanding, till the beginning of the twentieth century, Western medicine was not very popular in India. The colonial government started medical colleges along with Ayurvedic colleges and hospitals to popularize Western medicine. Many incentive schemes were introduced to attract people towards Western medicine. It was the discovery of penicillin and other *sulfa* drugs which were found effective in controlling many infectious diseases that the popularity and acceptance of Western medicine dramatically increased. Discoveries of vaccines for many life-threatening and disabling diseases established the superiority of Western over the indigenous systems. The ascendance of the modern medicine relegated Ayurvedic, folk and other systems of treatment and healing to a secondary status much before the independence of India in 1947.

In the independent India, Western (or modern) medicine was adopted as the official health care programme of the country. Striking decline in mortality and increase in lifespan in the last century led to the ascendance of modern medicine to this status. Rapid strides in surgical technology further contributed to the efficacy of modern medicine. It is accepted and promoted as the official health care system by almost all countries of the world. In India, more than 90 per cent of the national health budget is allocated for medical treatment. Health policies and programmes are primarily controlled by medical professionals, as is the highest governing body—Indian Medical Council. Both Ayurveda and folk healing are struggling to survive against the dominant status of modern medicine in public health care programme.

One of the criticisms of the indigenous system of medicine, particularly of Ayurvedic medicine is that these are not developed through the empirical method of clinical trials, as are the Western medicine (Zimmerman, 1999). Western medicines are approved to be used on human patients after their rigorous testing on primates and clinical samples. Ayurvedic medicines are refined and improvised through the trial-and-error method over many centuries. In Ayurveda, human body is considered to be the best laboratory and all new medicines are tried and tested on human patients. Ayurveda did not prescribe a standard medicine to all patients of a disease; the medicine varies according to the constitution and background of the patient. Lele (1986) comprehensively elaborated on the theoretical and scientific basis of Ayurveda and called upon the researchers and practitioners of Ayurveda to keep the efficacy of their treatment regimen using scientific methods. However, it is argued that had Ayurvedic practitioners intended to bring metaphysical view of life and society in their clinical practice, it would not have survived in the present scientific age. No practitioner of medicine, including Ayurvedic, can ignore learning from the clinical experiences to survive in the field.

Though, in present times, Ayurvedic medicines are proliferating in the market on the pattern of Western medicine. In 1964, the government set up an agency for setting norms for manufacture and control of the quality of traditional medicine. In 1970, the government of India passed the Indian Medical Central Council Act to standardize Ayurvedic teaching institutions, their curriculum and their diplomas. To promote traditional medicines, a scheme to appoint indigenous practitioners at primary and district health centres was implemented. The Department of AYUSH allocated funds to support research and develop traditional medicine and to set standards and regulate the activities related to practice of alternate systems of medicine.

In the cases of chronic diseases and preventive health care, the role of medical professionals is limited. Long-term health care and public and personal hygiene become important considerations in such cases. Indigenous health care systems with their holistic approach are more relevant in such cases. Indigenous systems brought health within the larger domain of socio-spiritual life of the person; health remained a social concern. With the cost of treatment rapidly escalating, medical treatment is neither viable nor affordable for a very large population of the world. Meeting the rising cost of treatment is becoming a serious problem in a developing country like India (Banerji, 2003).

We do not know at present how traditional systems of healing will survive and coexist with modern medicine in the time to come. Modern medicine is just hundred years old, whereas both Ayurveda and folk healing have been around for thousands of years. In their long history, both these systems of healing have gone through many existential crises and have survived. For the present, no clear pattern is discernible as to how they will survive in future. Modern medicine is promoted by all countries of the world at present as the scientific and advanced health care system. However, in last few decades, many serious shortcomings of modern medicine are discerned by patients, medical professionals and health researchers. Modern medicine by itself cannot meet all health needs of people and ensure their well-being (Cassell, 1991). As Khare (1996) has observed, people need both the medicine and God's grace to recover from an illness. A patient, therefore, seeks medical attention and at the same time prays for deliverance from the poor health condition. It may be interesting to watch how modern medicine will coexist as a system of health care along with the other existing systems. Alternative medicine and folk-healing systems are in crisis, but one can notice that their popularity graph has not declined. There are indications of the resurgence of indigenous systems and it will be interesting to watch how these indigenous systems of health and well-being will compete and complement modern medicine in the time to come.

3

Relevance of Faith Healing in the Scientific Age

The father of Western scientific medicine, Sir William Osler, wrote a classic paper in 1910 in the *British Medical Journal* entitled, 'The Faith That Heals.' In his article, Osler extolled many virtues of faith and its salutary role in health, healing and medicine. He concurred that faith is one of the miracles of human nature, which science is now ready to accept and also study its marvellous effects. It was this hope of the founding father of the Western medicine that research and practice of medicine would thrive on this human quality of faith. Sixty-five years later, American psychiatrist Jerome D. Frank revisited these themes in his paper by the same title 'The Faith That Heals' and agreed with Osler that faith "is an important topic that is conspicuously absent from the medical school curriculum" (1975, p. 127). In its pursuit to be scientific and objective, the Western medicine took a different root. Frank elaborated in his paper the significant implications which faith has for the healing of a patient, even if it has obvious religious overtones. Even 40 years after Frank's article, the scientific community in health and medicine is still debating how important is the consideration of 'faith' in recovering from a disease.

The critical significance of faith in health and healing was known in all traditional societies for ages. Based on the shared understanding of human nature and causes of suffering, these societies have developed their own healing institutions and practices. The faith healing systems so evolved independently in different parts of the world weathered the vagaries of time and have sustained (and thrived) in the present times on popular support. The works of Kleinman in East Asia and of Kakar in India are the testimonies to this fact. In India, a wide range of healers and healing centres, which include temples, *majārs*, shrines, local deities and so on are found in every nook and corner of the country. The burgeoning crowd which one sees around these places is a testimony to the fact that their relevance for healing the human psyche has not declined. Kakar (1982) has stated in his book, *Shamans, Mystics and Doctors*, that India is a country of healers. There are shamans, gurus, ojhas, *tantrics*, priests and faith healers, who specialize in dealing with a variety of social and personal problems. A gross estimate (VHAI, 1991) suggests that more than 90 per cent of the Indian population uses these services at some point in time. Nanda (2009) has presented evidence in her book, *The God Market*, that for 30 per cent of the population, faith in divine and spirituality has increased in the last five years. Thriving on folk wisdom and trusted by the masses, these faith-healing practices are still an enigma for the health scientists. The main objective of this paper is to examine faith healing as a viable system, its efficacy and acceptance in the scientific age.

The larger scientific community and modern medicine have remained critical and sceptical of the faith-healing practices. These are held as pre-scientific and considered to be practised by primitive and tribal people (Kothari & Mehta, 1988). It is further argued that ignorance and backwardness are primarily responsible for adherence to these non-scientific practices. But, as Watts (1975) contended, traditional healing practices are called primitive, mystical and esoteric because our education does not prepare us to comprehend their sophistication. Kakar (1982, 2003) and Kleinman (1980, 1988) have shown that most of these traditional practices are deeply entrenched in folk wisdom and time-tested theories of mind. They provide practical solutions to personal, familial and social problems, and have been integrated into the communal life for centuries. Despite their popular mass base, there is not enough work to test the premises of faith-healing practices on the scientific crucible. We need to decipher the folk wisdom and traditional knowledge behind the efficacy of faith healing (Dalal, 1991; Sheikh, Kunzendorf & Sheikh, 1989).

Faith healing thrives on the collective wisdom of a society, which is rooted in experience and practical considerations. Folk wisdom finds its expression in proverbs, folklores, legends, poetry, rituals and mythologies. These sources tell us how life problems are created, construed and controlled by the collective efforts of the community. In its struggle to maintain harmony and order, every society attempts to develop ecologically valid understanding of human nature; its own theories of suffering and remedial measures (Kleinman, 1988). In many anthropological texts (Mariott, 1955), faith-healing practices are considered within the little tradition, that is, the beliefs and practices of the masses. Shamans, spirits and local deities are all part of it. This is contrasted with the great tradition characterized by the practices based on classical and philosophical texts, such as the Vedas, the Upanishads and the Gita. In this, God is held as the Supreme Self, realized through contemplative meditation and devotional worships. It is a misconception that these two traditions are parallel and that the little tradition is subscribed by lower class and caste only. People who subscribe to faith healing belong to all strata of the society.

In India, faith-healing practices are, indeed, based on a complex and cohesive system of thoughts and beliefs, derived from philosophical texts and scriptures. Not only do such healing practices derive their legitimacy from the scriptures but also proved to be effective vehicles to translate the essence of scriptures in dialects that a common man can follow. It is, however, a contentious issue how folk wisdom and scriptures complement each other, in which folk wisdom got distilled and documented in classical texts, that in turn, has become a way of dealing with suffering in Indian society. Kakar has written extensively on faith healing and its relevance and efficacy in the last 40 years. His books (other than cited earlier)—*The Analyst and the Mystic* (1991), *Mad and Divine: Spirit and Psyche in the Modern World* (2008a), *Culture and Psyche: The Selected Essays* (2008b), *India Analysed: Sudhir Kakar in Conversation with Ramin Jahanbegloo* (2009) and many others have extensively dealt with faith and folk healing and their scientific import.

Faith healing is a message that how the mind can act as a healer for both mental and physical afflictions. The idea that the mind and the body are two aspects of the same reality and mutually influence each other has a long history in the West (Diaz, 1997). A close symbiotic relation between the mind and the body is accepted in the Indian tradition since ages. Therapists and healers know from their experience that the mind has powers to heal and their primary role is to activate this self-healing process. We still do not know much about how our emotions, expectations and anxieties turn into body's humeral and secretions which heal the body.

In the recent years, there is a resurgence of interest in understanding and acknowledging the contributions of these traditional practices in combating physical and mental illnesses. The limited success of the biomedical model and modern psychotherapies in the global scenario and their impersonal and market orientation has led to widespread discontentment. It is now widely accepted that psychotherapy works in the broader cultural context, which takes into consideration values and demands of the society (O'Hara, 2000). With the increase in stress-borne diseases and disorders, the spotlight is increasingly turning towards the age-old practices and examining their relevance in the modern world. There is a body of literature which concurs the intuitive understanding and cultural sensibilities which folk healers show about the working of the human mind and its potential to alleviate the suffering. This chapter explores the characteristic features of these healing practices and will attempt to decipher the way it works. The purpose is to draw parallels between folk practices and modern psychotherapies and identify learning opportunities from the ancient wisdom.

Proliferation of Healing Centres and Healers

Indigenous healing centres and healers can be found in every nook and corner of the country. There may be hardly any village in the country which does not have these healing centres. These places cover the whole range, from some temples or mosque to a shrine or an abode of a saintly figure. These are considered to be sacred places and are revered by its followers as places of worship. Many of these centres specialize in specific diseases and others are frequented by people of all faith, facing all kinds of life crises. There are individual faith practitioners called shamans or diviners or spiritual healers. They are believed to have miraculous powers to heal people afflicted by different diseases or disabilities.

Studies have shown that despite the progress of Western medicine and their availability everywhere, the popularity of the existing healing centres has not diminished. Faith healing is practised side by side with Western medicine as both religion and medicine are considered important to deal with health and illness. In India, most of these shamans and diviners hail from lower strata of the society and are often illiterate. Nevertheless, they are visited by rich and poor, educated and uneducated, professionals and daily wagers, alike. These shamans are not supposed to charge for their services. However, the prevalent view is that the quality of shamans has declined and they have become money-minded. There is also proliferation of healers and healing centres in recent times.

Three Faith-healing Centres

Three healing centres located in different regions of the country were visited by this author to examine how these healer centres function and heal people from physical and mental ailments. Two were faith-healing centres from Rajasthan near Udaipur and the third one was in the rural area of Allahabad. Enquiries were made about the people visiting these centres and how the healing takes place. These pilot studies also examined how the belief in supernatural facilitated recovery from the health problems.

Temple Healing of Paralytic Patients

First of these healing centres specializes in the treatment of paralysis and strokes. Located 40 km from Chittorgarh in Rajasthan in a picturesque valley and on the bank of a river, this place is an ideal location for outing in forests. Initially, it was a small temple of a local deity called *Avari Mata*. In the last three decades or so, this temple in the forest has grown into a small township with places to stay and eat.

The temple has a large courtyard, often packed with polio, paralysis and stroke patients and their families. Here, people come from many distant places and stay there till they show signs of recovery. They rent some place nearby and spend most of the day-time in the compound of the temple. Patients who go there mostly suffer from a paralytic attack, or other kind of impairment and immobility. In fact, as soon as people realize that they have been attacked by polio or paralysis, they rush to this temple town.

The place reverberates with hope and excitement. People keep arriving at any time of the day and night as the temple remains open 24 hours a day. They come with preparation to stay here for a longer period. Outside the courtyard of the temple, there is a vast stretch of open space along the river which people use for camping. They cook their food, gossip, play cards, chant *bhajans* (religious songs) and socialize with other visitors. Being away from home and daily routine, people look relaxed, free and enjoying the scenic surrounding. While sitting in small clusters, talking and sharing their health problem with each other, people often come to know about ways of dealing with the aftermath of a crisis, about the possibilities of treatment and leading a normal life. This mutual learning and sharing is the hallmark of their stay at the temple.

The patients who are brought to the temple premise do not just keep lying on their bed all the time. They are supposed to make *parikrama* (circumambulation) of the temple five times a day. This parikrama is not simply going round the temple. The tracking requires prostrating before the deity, walking a stretch, climbing a window, getting down at few other places and crawling through a narrow passage. The patients are helped by their family to complete the parikrama. My physiotherapist friend was of the opinion that this parikrama could be a good physiotherapy for the patients. People cry, plead and make offerings before the deity. All visitors assemble twice a day for puja and pray for their well-being. Those who can manage also go to the riverside to take a holy dip. The place looks very busy as something keeps happening there.

That the socio-spiritual therapy does work was evident from many narratives we took. In three to four days' time, the improvement in their health condition is for everyone to notice. Nima could not lift his left leg when he went there but went home walking after six days. For my medical friends, this is no mystery. Recovery in the cases of polio (though such cases have been rare for last 3–4 years) and paralytic stroke recovery at the initial stage is spontaneous and noticeable, even without any treatment. The temple ambience, faith and hope, the parikrama physiotherapy and mutual counselling contribute to the speedy recovery of the patients. The temple office for the last few years keeps a record of all visitors. In their record, they did not have a single case which did not improve. In reality, there might have been many, but nobody wanted to admit, including the patients who were not blessed by the Goddess.

Treatment of Affective Disorders

The second healing centre we had studied was located 20 km from Udaipur city in Rajasthan. It was the healing centre frequented by people with all types of physical, mental, family and work-related problems.

The place was better known for the treatment of affective disorders, especially hysteria, which in the local dialect is considered a problem of spirit possession, mostly inflicting women. In the local culture, hysteria, anxiety disorders, panic attacks and a host of other emotional pathologies are viewed as the instances of spirit possession. These are considered to be behavioural pathologies caused by some evil spirit possessing the patients. The local people take services of a diviner to drive away the evil spirit to restore selfhood of the person. Spirit possession is considered very normal, and there are usually set procedures for its treatment.

Women are generally more prone to such psychosomatic ailments. In the culture where women are subjugated and oppressed and feel constrained to vent out their pent-up feelings, these problems are common. There are the themes of harassment and torture of new brides by in-laws. These are the women who are ill-treated by their in-laws and find no support from husband and others. Their pent-up anger against the perpetrators keeps accumulating and they may find it increasingly difficult to cope with this onslaught on their person. Unable to handle the situation, many women break down and exhibit emotional and physical symptoms. Suffering from somatoform disorders, according to DSM-4, these women exhibit physical symptoms such as low back pain or limb paralysis, without apparent physical cause. The weird and unruly behaviour of such women is attributed to evil-spirit possession and prompts the family to consult a local healer (called ojha).

The place we visited was the healing centre of a local ojha, a small hut, a place to sit for 8–10 people, with photographs of many Gods, prominent being the monkey God Hanuman. The venue was on the periphery of a village, making it convenient for families of the afflicted women to visit the place for treatment. The diviner and the family, depending on the condition of the affected person, subjected him/her to a series of rituals and invocations aiming at driving away the evil spirit.

The day our team visited the place, a 22-year old married woman was brought there by the family. The woman was visibly not in her senses; she was crying and was abusive. Four family members had accompanied her, including her mother-in-law and brother-in-law. To drive away the evil spirit, the local healer asked the afflicted woman to sit on the altar, to prostrate before the deity and burnt a bunch of chillies close to her nose. The woman was visibly very uncomfortable and became abusive and started shouting. The healer asked her family members to hold her and engaged in chanting some mantras. Intermittently, he was yelling at the evil spirit to go away. The woman was becoming more unruly and for the healer, it was enough evidence that the evil spirit was volatile and was feeling threatened. The woman got exhausted and calmed down after a while. The family was asked to come back for another round of treatment on an appointed day.

On our next visit after few days, we got permission to talk to the afflicted woman. She was by now treated of the evil spirit and was apparently behaving normally. Her name was Shabari. She was the third daughter-in-law in a lower-middle-class joint family. Shabari's husband worked in Mumbai and visited her once in a year. Being the youngest daughter-in-law, she had to obey and serve her in-laws, including two elder sisters-in-law, who teased her constantly for her plain looks and poor parentage. Unable to bear it, she started getting fits of anger and during that spell, she would get abusive towards her sister-in-laws and would hurl stones at her father-in-law. Her family brought her to the healing centre to consult the diviner. In his state of trance, the diviner identified the spirit of an old woman which lived on the *peepal* tree (sacred fig) and had troubled three other women in the past. Shabari and her in-laws went through a series of elaborate rituals for the next few days. Finally, the diviner declared that the evil spirit has left Shabari. The family was asked to give alms to a needy one every Tuesday and observe certain rituals so that the evil spirit keeps away. We noticed that the attitude of in-laws towards Shabari was different this time. She was treated with little more respect by her family and community.

The cathartic value of spirit possession and consequent hostile behaviour of the patient is understandable. As a possessed woman, she was free to hurl abuses at her tormenters in the family, call them by names and even physically assault them. Her whole behaviour was likely to be attributed to the evil spirit possessing her. When her pent-up emotions were released, she was likely to feel lighter. This calming down of the patient was noticeable to all, with little trace of any unruly behaviour. She was shy of talking of what she was doing earlier and according to her she had no memory of how she was behaving. She was in her usual (even better) self as claimed by her in-laws, and attributed it to the monkey God whose grace helped her to be freed by the evil spirit. Much is written about the possession therapy and its healing consequences. Its scientific rationale is debatable. Its positive social-psychological consequences are acknowledged. Its consequences have to be seen in terms changing social

matrix in terms of relation of power, assertion and humanizing relationships (Kakar, 1982). Often, spirit possession is seen as another tool of
women's oppression in traditional societies, but alternatively, possession
encounters can be understood as a tool of empowering women and finding their legitimate place in the society. Equally important is the fact
that no stigma is attached to this mode of therapy, as one encounters in
the case of psychiatric treatment. Once the evil spirit has left, no one
blames the woman for her abusive and derogatory behaviour she had
indulged in under the spell.

The Snake Doctor

The third place I visited near Jodhpur, Rajasthan, was famous for the
treatment of snakebite. There was a shrine of Tejaji who died of snakebite. There is a legend that before Tejaji died, the snake gave him a boon
that any victim of snakebite paying homage at his shrine would be cured
of snakebite. There are many shrines of Tejaji in Rajasthan. I went to
one such shrine to watch how a snake doctor called *bhopa* treats the
cases of snakebite. It was a small temple in a desert area where one could
only see sand-dunes all around, far removed from human habitation.
The arid zone of Rajasthan is full of all kinds of snakes in summer, and
there are a number of snakebite cases every day. The anti-venom treatment is often available only in the city and it was not easy for everyone
to make it to the city, once bitten by the snake. I had visited the shrine
about 20 years back, but the scenario is only a little better now.

When I was at the shrine, a person bitten by a snake was brought in
a semi-conscious state. The bhopa checked the patient and the wound
and then planned his treatment according to his assessment of the seri-
ousness of the problem. He sat near the patient in a meditative posture
and then started reciting something while making strange gestures, as if
invoking some higher spirit, probably that of Tejaji. He had a fur baton
in his hand and kept hitting the patient with that while reciting something in a fast tone. I could not make out what he was chanting, nor
could of his strange behaviour. He pressed a long funnel on the open
wound and started sucking from the other end. He kept repeating the
same rituals many times while beating the patient with his fur baton.
It, of course, did not hurt the patient. The bhopa gave the impression

that he was bringing the patient back to his senses. To my amazement, the patient sat down after a while and after a half-an hour or so, walked back home without assistance. It was an amazing feat and I kept puzzling what cured him. Even a medical doctor would not have treated a patient of snakebite in such a short time. I was amazed.

I went to that healing shrine for the next four days and observed the bhopa treating six other patients of snakebite. Every time the result was more or less the same; the patients were walking back home at the end of the treatment.

I did not believe in miracles, but I did not understand what was happening. One day I happened to talk to one faculty in the Zoology Department of the University of Allahabad about this miraculous incident. He laughed at my ignorance. He told me that 80 per cent of the snakes in that region (and probably worldwide) are non-poisonous, and there are very few cases in which snakebite could be fatal. A sufficient quantum of the poison has to go into the blood stream for a person to die in the absence of the anti-venom treatment. So 80–90 per cent of the people bitten by a snake only need to be nursed for their wounds. What the faith healer was, in fact, doing was treating the patient of their acute anxiety and fears. The zoologist told me that there were cases when people not getting proper treatment died of snakebite and the post-mortem report showed that there was no poison in their bodies. They died of shock and intense fear, not due to the snake poison.

Obviously, the traditional healer was doing the psychological treatment of the patients of snakebite and saving at least 80 per cent of the lives, who if gone unattended, might have suffered serious health complications.

While reporting these findings, I am aware that there are quacks and cheats around, whose sole purpose is to fool the masses and make money. It is an issue which deserves an open debate. Most of the faith healers come from the lower strata of the society, and are poor and uneducated. It is very difficult to fix qualification for the faith healers who often follow their family tradition or learn the art of healing as an apprentice. Often the local people are able to discriminate who is a fake healer and who is not. For argument's sake, we can look at the medical data to gauge how many people die of wrong medication. In the world today, the medical profession is increasingly turning into a business where making money is the only goal. Faith healing is not immune to this malaise.

Community's Beliefs in the Supernatural

Social attitudes, beliefs, norms and values of a society provide the basis for making sense of symptoms, aetiology and import of any health problem. Meaning of social rituals, customs, communications, symbols and metaphors helps patients understand symptoms and implication of the disease in their life. The nature and intensity of suffering is understood in the holistic sense where events of the physical and social world only form the context and background.

Sharing the same culture, the healer and his/her healing practices are integral to the beliefs and practices of the local communities. The explanatory system which a healer employs is mostly congruous with the thinking of the community to which he or she belongs. Evolved over centuries, a wide cross section of Indian population believes in the supernatural powers of the healers and seeks their help for readdressal of the pain and suffering. These supernatural entities—local deity, Gods, ancestors, spirits, witches and demons—are all part of the socio-religious matrix of the community life. Their presence is invoked on many auspicious occasions as well as to ward off trouble and heal the suffering of the people. Some ancestors or spirits are more popular as kind and noble, and more easily accessible to the faith healers to treat people of various afflictions. In general, the theory of supernatural causation is widely believed and is frequently invoked to explain a wide range of events. Healing practices evolved around such beliefs have greater acceptability within communities, particularly in rural and tribal areas. Faith in healer and in his/her supernatural powers to heal is rooted in such belief system of the community.

Many of such community beliefs are considered false and delusional by the scientific community. These are attributed to superstition, illiteracy and ignorance prevalent among poor and rural people. The government, social activists and non-governmental organizations (NGOs) are called upon to educate people against false and illusionary beliefs. Such illusory beliefs about the prowess of faith healers are considered to be a major cause of the prevalence of backwardness and disease in the rural poor.

However, this position is contested even within the scientific community with research evidence that many such beliefs play a positive role in the recovery process and in adjusting to adverse life conditions.

Psychologists (Lazarus, 1983; Taylor, 1989) have reported positive consequences of many such 'illusory' beliefs and called them 'healthy illusions'. Hope and optimism may be 'unrealistic' but what they do to the psyche of a person is still a matter of serious investigation. Taylor (1889) and Wortman (1983) have shown that positively biased illusions are associated with and foster better life functioning as well as result in better health outcomes. This is counter to traditional theories of mental health in which reality perception is emphasized.

This debate to find which personal beliefs are real or true and which are illusionary or false could be endless, as beliefs, by definition, are not testable propositions. How can belief in God and supernatural be tested or how can one's faith in some person or group be subjected to verification? Faith and beliefs are often deep rooted, forming the basis of one's relation with self, family and community. How advisable it is to temper with them in the name of science and rationality is an agenda for a larger debate.

Why Faith Heals? A Western Perspective

Moerman et al. (1996, p. 141) reviewed the efficacy of faith on the basis of 17,000 studies taken from Medline search and reported that "it is regularly the case that 70% of patients can achieve good or excellent results with procedures subsequently shown to be ineffective in clinical trials." The review study clearly implicated the role of belief in God, worship and supernatural as having a therapeutic effect or, at least, contributing to the desired outcomes of medical therapy. It established that the faith heals.

Levin (2008) has tried to delineate as to how faith healing works. First, faith can heal by impelling the person to engage in healthy behaviour that strengthens the body's immune system and by preventing the person from indulging in negative behaviour. Second, faith can heal by connecting one to like-minded people who can offer tangible and emotional support and encouragement. Particularly, sharing and confiding to own group can ameliorate stress and moderate its deleterious effects on human physiology. Third, faith can heal by establishing a thinking pattern that affirms one's innate healing ability. It could be grounded in our beliefs in supernatural acquired in early life as a member of a community. Fourth, faith can heal by engendering positive emotions through personal or community-related beliefs, thoughts and experiences. Fifth, faith can heal by reinforcing hope for a better future and enhancing pain tolerance. It may enhance self-regulation of physiological functioning. The belief and trust implicit in expressions of religious faith are consonant with mental actions necessary for desired bodily responses.

Ambience of the Healing Centres

In spite of many studies and publications in this area in the last 2–3 decades, our understanding of how faith healing works is very limited. There is a large body of evidence that the faith works, but what actually happens in the process of faith healing that leads to both mental and physical recovery of the faith is still an enigma. Does the faith work in the same manner as in the doctor's chamber, as in a dilapidated hutment of a village healer? There is evidence that a medical physician's prescription may not work if the patient had little trust in the doctor or in the medicine prescribed (Koenig, 1999; Mechanic and Schlesinger, 1996).

Talking about the Indian rural scenario, it is a general observation that the healing sessions do not take place in the private chambers of the healers, where there is one-to-one communication between the healer and the client. It takes place in an open ground or in a hall which is accessible to everyone. Healing is taken as a social activity, where besides the healer and the patients, there are family members of the patients, neighbours and other villagers who assemble to witness the healing process. People share their problems and consult the healer in full public view. Families and other community members are not silent spectators but actively indulge in the treatment process by adding to the story of the patients and their families, even contradicting what was said. Everybody knows everyone's problem and it becomes a participatory venture to help out the afflicted person.

This kind of ethos is ideal for the social construction of a problem and its remedy which has the approval and acceptance of the community. These are the places where a personal problem is no longer seen from the egocentric perspective but within the larger social framework. Participation in social ritual and social nature of healing activities helps in relocating the person on a larger social canvas. This shift in focus from personal to social is important for relocating the ailing person within the social matrix.

Faith healing is holistic in nature. It focuses on the person, not on the specific problem one is suffering from. In healing sessions, the attention on the problem is only peripheral; the emphasis is on 'who is suffering'? These are the people, not the 'patients', who are helped to regain their normal functioning. The healers often belong to the same region and know the family background and history of the patient's problem. Their concern is to alleviate the suffering of the patients. As stated by Kleinman (1988), in all Asian cultures, body-self is not a secularized private domain of the individual person, but an organic part of the sacred, socio-centric world, a communication system involving the exchange with others, including the divine.

These faith healers know intuitively or from their experience that mind and body are closely intertwined. The body cannot remain healthy when the mind is sick and vice versa. The healer creates conditions in which physiological processes are connected with meaning and relationships so that patient's social world is linked recursively to one's inner experiences. In the case of a health problem, the ailing person has a tendency to withdraw from the social world into their own ego-shell and remain uncommunicative to their larger social world. Faith healing reverses this process.

Faith-healing centres are considered to be the sacred places. These could be temples, majārs, tomb, a holy tree, shrine of a saint or an open place considered to be sacred. Across the length and breadth of the country, there is no dearth of places which are known for their healing powers. Different healing practices use different forms of sacred, but for most of them, the physical and metaphysical worlds overlap. Deities, demons and spirits are as much part of this physical world as they are of the metaphysical. Faith healing engages them in the healing process, and bringing harmony between these two worlds is one of the objectives of healing rituals. The sacredness of these places is maintained by the priests, swamis, fakirs, tantrics and gurus who manage these places. It may also be mentioned here that though sacred, many of these healing centres are secular and thronged by the believers of different faiths.

The sacredness of the healing practices is further reinforced by the legends associated with the healer and/or healing centre. The author surveyed 18 such shrines in Uttar Pradesh and Rajasthan, famous for their healing prowess. Each one of these centres had a story about how that shrine came into existence. It was either a deity who instructed a devotee in the dream, some paranormal phenomena observed on a particular spot, miraculous recovery near some enchanted grooves, deification of a sati or boon bestowed on a devotee to have supernatural powers. These legends of derived powers are recounted with reverence by the visitors, who often know these healing stories by heart.

Invariably, at a faith-healing centre, even when the healer is operating independently, there are pictures of Gods, deities or local legends. Their benevolence and grace are believed to be important for the well-being of the suffering individual. The place is often suffused by the flagrance of essences which are profusely lit to create an aura of mysticism. Sometimes along with the essences, smokescreen is created by burning some local stuff (called *gugul* in northern India). Other rituals are performed to invoke some desired spirit. The whole atmosphere is charged with reverence and awe in which people who had gathered wait with heightened expectation something paranormal to occur.

The faith healers often belong to the same clan and subscribe to the same belief system as that of their clients. Often, they are not formally educated to practice their art but learn it through apprenticeship and assisting their gurus. Many of them inherit their right to practice and this may be a prerogative of few families whose members are presumed to possess special powers to heal. No matter what is the background of these healers, they need long years of internal preparation to acquire purity of body and mind. As observed by Kakar (2003), it is the matter of unquestioned faith in the paranormal powers of the healer which is at the core of all positive outcomes. It is the belief in the person of the healer, not his or her conceptual system or specific technique which is of decisive importance in the healing process. What is of prime importance is the trust and confidence that a healer is capable of instilling in the minds of its clientele. The aura and authority of a healer are carefully cultivated through the stories of miraculous healing.

These faith healers are often considered to be mediators between the physical and the metaphysical. They are supposed to acquire the ability to host a deity or spirit, under whose spell they acquire supernatural powers to control minds of the visitors and heal them. The healer becomes the medium through which others can communicate to deities and spirits. Under the spell of a deity or some other noble spirit, healers acquire visions, can read patients' mind and tell them what will heal them. As they transform into diviners during the healing sessions, these healers are presumed to be in direct communication with the supernatural and derive their healing powers through divine grace. They are both feared and revered by the local communities. Of course, they become diviners only on the occasions when possessed by some spirit. Other times, they are like any other person in the community.

Faith-healing Sessions

While discussing what happens in a healing session, it should be clear that mostly there is no uniform procedure of healing which a healer follows. The cultural diversity of the country has facilitated the growth of diverse practices in different regions. These faith therapies differ not only in terms of rituals but also in terms of their sophistication and belief system. However, there are no fixed procedures which the healers follow in their dealing with the patients. Even the same healer does not follow the procedure every time. There is a great deal of spontaneity in the way healing rituals are performed. At all the places I visited, informal environment pervaded in which everyone was free to opine and actively participate. There were some rituals which were sacrosanct, and were to be performed properly; the supernatural had to be given its due respect and any sacrilege is not tolerated. Most of the other ceremonies and procedures were flexible and depending on other considerations and constraints, healing rituals are added, deleted or modified on a particular day or for a particular patient. There is rarely any elaborate planning before the healing session. People, who assemble laugh, make fun, mock at each other, smoke and comment and enjoy being there. In this scenario, it is a daunting task for any social scientist to capture the range and diversity of these healing practices and to conjecture how they work.

Of course, in the healing session, it is the healer who regulates the proceeding and takes the centre stage. The faith healers have no training in hypnosis but master the art of heightening people's suggestibility to induce a particular type of imageries and healing messages. Besides burning essence and gugul to create opaqueness, there are other techniques which the faith practitioners employ to alter mental state of the affected people, such as chanting, slow breathing, rhythmic dancing, fasting, sensory and social isolation and so on. These group and other activities facilitate lulling of the conscious mind, rendering the unconscious mind more receptive to positive imageries induced by the healer. The subliminal messages transacted through may have a powerful influence on the person.

The main focus in healing session is on the exchange between the healer and the suffering individual. Whatever be the affliction, there are emotional distress and symptoms of anxiety, fear, withdrawal, dissociation and so on. These symptoms further aggravate the suffering individual's physical and mental functioning. An experienced healer knows that these people need reassurance. A healer creates an aura of authority over the natural and supernatural and reinforces the belief of a sufferer and her family that he can control the course of tragic events. For this, it is not very important what kind of verbal exchange takes place between the two, but how effectively the non-verbal messages are put across and received. The healing rituals facilitate transmission of healing messages through the extensive use of cultural symbolism. Many of the rituals are of social nature in which family and other members of the community also join. These rituals serve the purpose of reconnecting the suffering person to his/her social network. Directly or indirectly, such people tend to develop a sense of belonging and learn to situate their problem in the larger social matrix.

This process of reconnecting with the metaphysical becomes more intense in the situation where the healer is possessed by a deity or some noble spirit, who communicates to the sufferer. This communication often has a salutary effect on the person who feels now reassured of his/her well-being and calms down. In the beginning of such spell, there is much commotion in which the ailing person presumed to be possessed by some evil spirit shows all kinds of weird behaviour, shouts, cries, accuses and uses filthy language. Nobody takes an offence as it is believed to be doings of the evil spirit. The audience is witness to this clash of evil spirit and self of the person. Once this spell is over, the order is restored at the healing place. This, of course, does not happen in the case of every person who comes for healing. However, in general, it is the tremendous outpouring and channelizing of patients' emotions and faith which seem to be responsible for dramatic improvement in their condition. Chanting bhajan in a chorus is an example of emotional outpouring.

Faith-healing practices achieve positive outcomes by focusing on changing unhealthy patterns of thinking, feeling and behaving and prepare the person to face the vicissitudes of the problems in their social world. At times, the actual problem may not go away but as a consequence of the faith therapy, people learn to live with it. This therapy soothes the troubled ego of the person. In other words, the therapy may result in (a) symptom relief and (b) improved functioning. Symptom relief is achieved by lowering expectations, whereas improved functioning is contingent on remodelled pattern of social interaction for which others in the family have to change as well. The ambience, rituals and activities at the healing place foster this coming back of the suffering person to the social fold. Imposition of social meaning on one's illness and exposure to cultural symbolism brings the person face to face with others in the society and participation in the healing rituals implies that the person is accepted as equals by those who matter in the community. Healing occurs through the broadening of the network of relationships (Kapoor, 2003). Community healing marks the transition of a person from personal to social identity.

In Indian communities, faith healers know from their personal experience that treating the ailing person is not enough. Unless the family and the community to which the person belongs change, any improvement in the mental health will be short lived. Very often, the problems for which people come to a healer have its genesis in unhealthy social relationships. It is, therefore, imperative that all concerned parties participate in the healing process. This open system of healing creates space for everyone to join and participate, which in turn is a learning experience for the whole community.

In the case of hysterical outbursts as we observed at one healing centre, what was gratifying for the ailing woman was change in the family's attitude. It was as if the whole family woke up to her existence and were paying attention to her needs and welfare. Many women reported that after their recovery, the family was treating them more gently for the fear of the local deity. The family and other relatives who participate in the healing rituals, many of which take place in the home setting, are directed to bring about attitudinal change. Most of these activities are not systematically planned by the healer, nor are explicitly targeted at the family. This flexibility in the healing practices leaves enough scope for innovation.

What is being discussed here is based on social science perspective and is tentative. Our knowledge of how faith therapies work is rudimentary as there is a real dearth of empirical studies to throw light on the process and mechanism underlying such healing.

Faith Healing in the Age of Science

How is faith healing seen in the present time? There is no answer to this question, but there are three alternative ways in which faith healing is constructed. A view which was formulated by the Western medical anthropologists in the early part of the last decade is the magico-religious system of healing. Western anthropologists, who studied Asian and African indigenous healing practices, termed them as magico-religious (see Hewson, 1998; Leslie, 1998). It is supposed to be practised by those who hail from poor, uneducated, primitive and subaltern sections of the society. Their world view and social life are presumed to be governed by their customs and beliefs whose legitimacy lies in religion and miracles. These people are presumed to live in a make-believe world where healers create an illusion of treatment by their magical powers. It is widely believed that their healing practices are based on superstition, false beliefs and blind faith. In India also, many of the tribal and subaltern healing practices are seen as magico-religious, not grounded in the reality (Dalal, 2000a).

The second view considers the efficacy of faith healing as placebo effect. The subscribers of this view do not deny the fact that faith healing works in many instances but attribute it to the time factor. WHO Annual report of 1998 clearly states that 80 per cent of the diseases we suffer from are of self-limiting nature, that is, either have fix duration or taken care by the body's healing system. The point is that no medication is required in a large number of disease conditions. Many times in medical practices, placebo drugs which have no chemical agent (like sugar pills or vitamin tablets) are prescribed by the doctors, when the health problem is seasonal or disease is of mild nature. Erwin (1959) emphatically argued with support that about 65–70 per cent improve after treatment regardless of the type of treatment. There are a number of studies where placebo drugs were found as effective as standard drugs. For example, the efficacy of Prozac could not be distinguished from placebo in six out of ten clinical trials (Moore, 1998). Placebos are also known as make-believe drugs (Burne, 2002). Faith healing is also held as a kind of placebo effect which, in essence, has no ingredient to heal and, therefore, as far as recovery of the patient is concerned (Miller, Colloca & Kaptchuk, 2009).

The third view takes faith healing more seriously and considers it as an active agent in the healing of the person (Frank & Frank, 1991). Faith healing is found to accentuate hope and expectations, activate body's immune system and energize the ailing person to actively participate in the recovery process. The holistic nature of the faith therapy facilitates readjustment in becoming an active and productive member of the community. Faith healing in this sense is a system of health intervention, like other psychotherapeutic interventions. As concluded by Levin (2008), the healing power of faith is notable on account of three defining characteristics: (a) it is naturalistic, (b) it is consistent with current scientific understandings of mind–body interaction and (c) it does not require belief in any supernatural agency. However, faith in supernatural accentuates the efficacy of faith healing in many instances (Vanderpool, 1977). What is important is that faith and beliefs create conducive mental state to facilitate bodily recovery of patients. There is now a substantial body of research evidence to argue that what we consider as ignorance and superstitions are, in fact, significant psychological resources for patients.

The growing popularity of faith healing is a testimony to the fact that it works. Faith healing has been around for thousands of years and is still practised all over the world, not by primitive societies but all sections of the society. It is unfortunate that psychology and medical science have not paid sufficient emphasis of research in this area. What is known to be a simple folk healing in a village in India is still considered an enigma and superstition by the academic and scientific community. We need to develop conceptual and methodological tools to establish a causal connection between folk-healing practices and the well-being of the targeted person. Research in this area would hopefully help us in understanding the hidden powers of mind to heal and improve well-being of human societies.

4

Integrating Traditional Services within Primary Health Care

India's present health care planning is primarily based on the Western medical model. Medical and mental health care practices are cast in Western theories and therapeutic practices. The medical model has dictated health care planning, policies and programmes all these years after the independence of India from the British rule. In the last Five Year Plan (Draft Report, 2013), about 97.3 per cent of India's health care budget was allocated to modern medicine; in the rest, all other alternative systems of medicine were covered. Governmental and other regulatory bodies are dominated by medical doctors. In spite of tall claims of looking at the health from a broader perspective, it is the disease model which is at the core of India's health care services.

In the past two decades, a major shift in the health care has taken towards privatization. The *India Health Report* (Confederation of Indian Industry, 2010) states that the contribution of the private sector in terms of the availability of hospital beds has gradually increased from about 28 per cent in 1973 to about 61 per cent in 1996. The report estimates this number to be 78 per cent in 2009. A more recent Indian Health Care Sector Report (Draft Report, 2014) shows that 80 per cent medical doctors work in private hospitals. Various incentive schemes of the government, such as tax exemptions, subsidized allocation of land, income tax rebate, incentives for privatization of medical education and easy availability of public finance has led to rapid growth of private hospitals. The provision of 100 per cent foreign direct investment (FDI) in the health sector has led to massive investment from international financial corporations, including the World Bank. As the draft plan of the National Health Policy 2015 shows, in 2012–1213 alone, private health care industry has attracted over 2 billion dollars of FDI. A natural offshoot of this privatization is the development of super-speciality medical centres in the metropolitan India. These super-specialty centres are comparable to the best known centres in the worlds. As a result, India has become a much sought after destination for medical tourism by the patients of Western countries. Confederation of Indian Industry (ASSOCHAM Report, 2011) reported on the basis of feedback from the organization's member hospitals that 150,000 medical tourists came to India in 2005. The number grew to 200,000 by 2008. It estimated that in the last decade, 850,000 medical tourists came to India and projected that by 2015, the number of foreign patients visiting India would rise to 3,200,000 (Press Release, ASSOCHAM Report, 2011). These figures were corroborated by the McKinsey and Company Report (May, 2008) which observed that India had 150,000 medical tourists from the United States in 2002 which increased to 450,000 in 2007. There is a phenomenal increase in medical tourists from other developed countries as well as patients from neighbouring countries. One reason for India to be such a favoured destination for orthopaedic and heart problems is that the cost is only 25 per cent of what would the insurance companies pay in the United States for the same quality of treatment. India has become a booming health care industry. A small town of Noida, near Delhi, is emerging as a hotspot for medical tourism. A number of hospitals have hired language translators to make patients from Balkan and African countries feel more comfortable in communicating with the medical staff. The city of Chennai has been termed as India's health capital with a large number of multi-speciality and super-specialty hospitals bringing in an estimated 150 international patients every day.

Health is thus increasingly reduced to an industry from a service sector. A public service has been transformed into a for-profit enterprise in which physicians are 'health care providers', serving the interest of big corporate, and patients are reduced to consumers. A service sector that it was, medicine is now converted into a business with deprofessionalized doctors and far worse, depersonalized patients. This radical change in medical practices in past 25–30 years has transformed a healing profession increasingly into an industry run by technicians. The health care scene is dotted by super-specialty, cutting-edge technology and tertiary care, where the patients are simply reduced to consumers. This health industry is thriving on affluent, highly insured and influential Indians who could afford the exorbitant cost of medical treatment.

It is ironical that this is happening in a country which lacks basic infrastructure for primary health care to reach out its larger population. Health care services are increasingly getting out of bounds of those who are poor and cannot pay for expensive private treatment. Governments after governments have let the public health services decay and become almost defunct over the decay. There is no larger debate about what health care implies and how these services can effectively reach the masses. We need to rethink our priorities and deliberate on the alternate model of health care which is compatible with our rich heritage, social expectations and contemporary developments. As Evan Ellich (1974) stated almost 40 years back that health care decisions cannot be solely left in the hands of medical professionals (or industry), but needs the wider participation of all stakeholders. We need to deliberate on viable models of health care to reach out to all cross sections of people.

Dismal Scenario of Public Health Care

The scenario looks bleak when we view the state of public health care services which cater to 80–85 per cent of the poor Indians who mostly reside in rural areas or urban slums. This overwhelmingly large population has no financial resources to access private hospitals. One must view India's health care scenario keeping in mind the fact that India's 42 per cent of the population (456 million people) lives below the revised poverty line (income below $1.25 a day) (World Bank Report, 2008). A majority of this population lives in rural areas where medical care is scarce and inaccessible. With limited men and monetary resources and crumbling infrastructure, it seems impossible for the government to provide even minimum health care services to its citizens.

The pathetic state of public health care is creating havoc in the life of a common man. The *India Health Report*, released by the Confederation of Indian Industry (CII) in 2010 has pointed out that there is a critical gap in the need and availability of infrastructure in terms of sheer health care sub-centres and trained staff even if the quality is not considered.

This inadequate access to quality health care is particularly deleterious for the poor, lower caste, rural people and women. According to the Report, about 7–8 per cent of households are pushed below the poverty line because of expenses incurred on health care. National data reveal that 50 per cent of the bottom quintile sold assets or took loans to access private hospital care. In fact, a nationwide survey of medical expenditure conducted by the National Council of Applied Economic Research revealed that among the poor, expenditure incurred to meet the medical needs is the second most important cause of rural indebtedness after daughter's marriage (Banerji, 2003). Another study showed that in India, 80 per cent of the health care expenses are borne by the users, 90 per cent of which are by the poor people (Krishnakumar, 2004). This scenario is corroborated by many recent health surveys. An extensive primary health care infrastructure turned inadequate because of the dismal quality of care it provided to the India's poor (Bajpai & Goyal, 2004).

Instead of improving the quality and efficiency of public health care system, the government focused on providing health insurance to the poor people. For example, Rajiv Aarogyasri Health Insurance Scheme (RAHIS) was introduced in various states in 2007. This scheme looked good on paper, but not necessarily reducing health expenditure or improving health conditions of the Indian masses. It was found to increase the revenue source of corporate hospitals. One recently conducted household survey in Andhra Pradesh by ACCESS International (Project Report, 2014) showed an overall reduction in out-of-pocket expenditure but had limited impact on rural indebtedness among the two lowest quintile groups. In 2013–2014, the government introduced health insurance scheme for those who are below poverty line. They are given insurance coverage of ₹30,000 per annum per family. The new central government increased the insurance amount to 100,000 rupees, covering about the population of 370 million in 2014 (National Health Policy, 2015). It is hoped that with health insurance coverage of such a vast population, the private investment will move in the direction of creating health care facilities for the poor. The expectations are rife that instead of investing only in tertiary and super-speciality services in urban areas, private finance may move in the direction of opening quality hospitals in the rural areas. In any case, improving the quality of public health care services, especially of primary health centres, still remains a distant dream

Universal Health Care in India: A Chronology of Expansion

In the last 68 years of independence, India has many achievements in the health sector. In fact, all health indicators registered an improvement over this period. We have been able to completely eradicate smallpox and polio and reduce the incidences of leprosy, TB, AIDS and other communicable diseases. The infant mortality rate (IMR) has come down by 2015 from a high of 110 in 1981 to 68 in 2000 and to 42, maternal mortality rate 560 in 1990 to 141, the total fertility rate of 2.4 which is getting closure to replacement rate of 2.1, though it is at the cost of declining female sex ratio (estimate, National Health Policy draft, 2015). These figures are still very high, vis-à-vis other countries at comparable or even lower levels of development. As a result, the overall life expectancy at birth has doubled from 32.4 years in 1951 to 64.7 years for male and 68.3 years for females by 2014 (Human Development Report, 2014). These average life expectancy figures for India hide a great deal of variation in the performance of different states. While Kerala, Maharashtra and Tamil Nadu are doing better, the states of Odisha, West Bengal, Bihar, Rajasthan, Madhya Pradesh and Uttar Pradesh are way behind.

In 1978, India became a signatory to the Declaration of Alma-Ata acknowledging health as a fundamental human right and focusing on primary health care to provide universal care to all citizens. According to this declaration, primary health care was to have its base in the community it serves. The primary health care included maternal and child care, family planning, immunization for major infectious diseases, prevention and control of locally endemic diseases, appropriate treatment of common diseases and injuries, provision of essential drugs, education concerning prevailing health problems and ways to deal with them, provision of adequate food and nutrition and adequate supply of clean water. The Declaration of Alma-Ata set a goal for the year 2000 for all the people of the world to achieve a level of health such as to enable them to lead socially and economically productive lives. Expansion of primary health care infrastructure and services became a major objective of India's health planning. Primary health care is provided through a network of sub-centres, primary health care centres, community health centres and district hospitals. In rural areas, primary health care is mostly provided by sub-centres or primary health centres; whereas in urban areas, it is provided via health posts and family welfare centres.

In 1982, when the government reformulated National Health Policy and officially adopted the WHO declaration of 'Health for All by 2000', many significant changes were made at the policy level (Chatterjee, 1993). The new policy envisaged a role for local communities and for social sciences in promoting public health care. The new National Health Policy put greater emphasis on rural health infrastructure development which became a major thrust area for the government in the 1980s and 1990s.

Remarkable progress was made in those two decades in health infrastructure development. Infrastructure for rural health was build up with a massive expansion of sub-health centres and Primary Health Centres (PHCs), with emphasis on maternal and child care, family welfare and hygiene education. To develop a network of health care centres, the Indian government set the following targets: one sub-centre with one trained female and one trained male health worker per 5,000 persons in the plains and per 3,000 persons in hilly and tribal areas. One PHC staffed by a medical officer and other paramedical staff per 30,000 persons in the plains and 20,000 persons in hilly, tribal and backward areas. Each PHC was to supervise six sub-centres. One community health centre (CHC) or upgraded PHC with 30 beds and other basic facilities per 80,000–120,000 persons. The CHC is to operate as a referral centre for up to four PHCs. As a result of this massive expansion by 1998, there were 137,006 sub-centres, 23,179 PHCs and 2,913 CHCs in India. There were 665,639 hospital beds or 6.9 hospital beds per 10,000 persons. In terms of manpower planning, a remarkable achievement was the training of 400,000 of community health workers (CHWs) within five years (1977–1982), almost one CHW for each village in the country, constituting the largest health care cadre in the world. This expansion was so rapid that the targets of developing infrastructure by 2000 were met in 1991 itself (Chatterjee, 1993).

However, such massive expansion was not enough to provide health care to all citizens. The National Family Health Survey II (NFHS II, 1998–1999) revealed that in terms of coverage, only 13 per cent of rural residents had access to a PHC, 33 per cent had access to a sub-centre, 9.6 per cent had access to a hospital and 28.3 per cent had access to a dispensary or clinic. One of the major determinants of the use of a health care facility, wherever they exist in reality, is the distance to the location of the facility from the user's home. This is especially true for women and children in rural areas. Overall, 47.4 per cent villages had access to any health facility within their village and 38.9 per cent villages had access to any facility within less than 5 km. Thus, the existing extensive network of public health centres fell far short both in terms of population coverage as per the guidelines set out by the government. The poor being the main users of primary health care facilities, the rich preferring to use private clinics and hospitals, the absence of public primary health care services means that many people either forego any medical care altogether or use too little, too late or choose to seek expensive and unregulated care in the private sector. Indigenous and alternative medicines were kept out of these primary health care services.

In the 1990s, a major shift in the national health policy took place in which management of PHCs and sub-centres were turned over to local self-governments, the Panchayati Raj. Initially, there was a lot of enthusiasm and hope that it will make health services more accountable to local communities. But, like many other schemes, it also got mired in many controversies and rarely showed the desired results. Panchayats in India are not a true representative of the people but are dominated by the powerful elite and power brokers. In the feudal system that still prevails in rural India, decentralization and bottom-up approach rarely succeed. It is anachronistic to the prevailing ethos and functioning of the government.

In 2002, the government announced a new health policy with the main objective of achieving an acceptable standard of good health of the general population. The policy aimed to strengthen the infrastructure, decentralize health care delivery through Panchayati Raj, setting up national accounting services and to regulate the private practice. These were all laudable goals but no proper mechanism was worked out to implement the provisions of this policy. In fact, this new policy was a kind of rundown for the already depleted primary health centres. The new policy ignored the earlier health policy's objectives of providing primary health care for all, especially to the underprivileged (Qadeer, 2001). The commitment of the earlier policy to create a well-worked out referral system was dumped to make way for privatization and commercialization of health services. The government opened up the health sector for the private enterprises in a hope that with better monitoring and regulations, the private sector will ease resource crunch in the health sector.

As a follow up of the National Health Policy 2002, the National Rural Health Mission (NRHM) was launched in 2005 with the objective of providing accessible and affordable quality health care to the rural population. It sought to re-invigorate the system of health care by bringing about architectural correction in the health systems. It adopted the following main strategies: increased involvement of communities in planning and management of health care facility, improved programme management, flexible financing and provision of untied grants, decentralized planning and augmentation of human resources. It provides special focus on 18 states, which have weak public health indicators and weak infrastructure. In terms of systems improvements, the NRHM targets were the upgradation of all PHCs into 24 × 7 PHCs by the year 2010 and upgrading all CHCs to Indian Public Health Standards and engagement of 400,000 female Accredited Social Health Activists (ASHAs) in providing the first-level health services to village women.

The Present Scenario

Many commentaries and critics are of the opinion that India's health care system itself is critically sick and in intensive care unit (ICU). An Independent Commission on Health in India, which submitted its report to the former Prime Minister Mr Vajpayee, pointed out that the health services are in an 'advanced stage of decay'. Documents from the Planning Commission paint an equally dismal picture (Planning Commission of India, 2004). This scenario has worsened in the last one decade.

In most of the rural sector, PHCs are barely surviving or are non-existent, in spite of all pronounced policies, programmes and financial support of the government. The quality of health care services provided by the public health system is extremely low along all the criteria on which quality can be judged—infrastructure, availability of drugs and equipment, regular presence of qualified medical personnel and treatment facilities for the patients. Instead of being supportive and palliative of people's health, it will not be wrong to say that the health care system itself poses a hazard to its intended beneficiaries, especially the poor, who are often as reluctant to use public health services as the rich people are.

One notable failure of most of the rural health programmes is low community participation. Imposed from outside by the government functionaries and NGOs, these programmes could not garner community support. Western and westernized NGOs are incompatible with local culture, needs and aspirations of people. Local health practices and resources were not taken cognizance of, nor were services of traditional practitioners acknowledged.

One of the major lacunae in India's health system in India is that there is no effective monitoring system. There is no proper public readdressal mechanism to ensure appropriate standards of care in clinical practices. This is equally true of the public as well as private sectors which are largely unregulated. The Medical Council of India, the apex body overseeing standards of care, has no process in place whereby doctors are assessed for their competence to deliver quality services according to set norms. The renewal of doctors' registration is mostly a routine procedure. Given the lack of effective monitoring, there is little information to go by in terms of competence of medical personnel and actual practice in a clinical setting; though there is substantial evidence of overuse of antibiotics and tranquilizers in public health care centres (Harihar, 2012).

Delivery of public health care services in India is marked by pervasive absenteeism. According to a study, absenteeism among doctors was as high as 43 per cent and among other health workers, 39 per cent in government health care facilities across Indian states (Chaudhury et al., 2006). A survey conducted by Banerjee (2000) in Udaipur in Rajasthan found greater absenteeism in PHCs and CHCs than in sub-centres. This meant that for people seeking health care services, there was considerable uncertainty attached to a visit that is costly in terms of time and travel expenses. On arrival at a PHC, there is no guarantee that it will be open on working days; if open, will there be a doctor and other staff around. Such uncertainty further attenuates people's motivation to make use of public health facilities. Under the family welfare programme, health and family planning workers are required to make regular visits to each household in their assigned area to monitor women and children's health, to provide family planning information and counsel and deliver selected services. Only 13 per cent of women in India, according to the NFHS II (1998–1999), reported receiving a visit from a health or family planning worker in the last 12 months preceding the survey.

Apart from absenteeism of the medical and paramedical staff in the rural areas, another problem is the high staff shortage. There is a shortage of 85 per cent specialist doctors, 75 per cent medical doctors,

80 per cent lab technicians, 53 per cent nursing and 52 per cent ANMs in government facilities across the country. Medical personnel prefer to work in private hospitals and that too in the bigger cities. As a result, the rural services stay defunct where the villagers have to visit city nursing homes and private hospitals for treatment. This scenario needs to be viewed in the light of the fact that India has 355 medical colleges from which annually 440,000 doctors and 22,000 specialist graduates pass out; 290 dental colleges with annual turnover of 21,000 dentists; 2,400 nursing schools and 1,500 colleges from which 1.2 lakh nurses pass out; in addition to 30,000 auxiliary nurse midwives and 70,500 pharmacists getting trained every year (National Medical Statistics, 2013). Most of them are concentrated in towns and cities in private set-ups. The government has not been able to deal with the crisis of staff shortage.

Doctor–Patient Communication

For proper diagnosis and deciding about treatment regimen, doctor–patient communication is crucial. In India, there are vast sub-cultural differences between the doctor and the patient which affect their mode and content of communication. Quite often medical practitioners learn from their personal experiences that diagnosis would be more accurate and treatment would be more beneficial if patient's socio-economic background, beliefs, needs and anxieties are taken into consideration, along with the biological status. Nevertheless, it is presumed that the patient would be receptive, willing to furnish necessary information and conform to the treatment regimen. It may be so in the case of hospitalized patients. In cases of chronic diseases particularly, patients and their families do not always accept the passive role and frequently engage in 'secret forms of curing' depending on their appraisal of the disease and its course. This is universally true, more so in the case of traditional societies. It is thus important to view doctor–patient communication in the Indian cultural setting, particularly in the context of biomedical treatment (Jayasunder, 2012).

In the crowded Indian hospitals where the ratio of doctor to patients is dismally low, no ideal pattern of doctor–patient communication can be achieved. Due to acute shortage of medical doctors in the government hospitals, there is always an unending stream of patients which a doctor has to attend. The doctor cannot spare much time for the individual patients and as a consequence, the communication is largely confined to patient symptoms and writing a medical prescription for some diagnostic tests or medication. The doctor has no time to hear about the patients' problems in detail and as a consequence patients, by and large, are dissatisfied with their communication with the doctor.

In India, medical doctors and patients come from a different socio-economic background. Doctors are mostly from higher castes and from economically well-off background, who can afford expensive medical education. The few who come from lower castes are those whose families have already moved upward economically. On the contrary, most of the patients in government dispensaries are those who belong to lower strata of the society. More than 86 per cent of the patients in India are poor and cannot afford expensive treatment in private hospitals and specialty centres. They get the raw deal as treatment facilities at primary health centres are almost non-existent.

Doctors and patients in India not only belong to different social classes but also have a different interpretation of the disease, particularly about its causality. Doctors trained in biomedicine often explain diseases in term of viruses and bacteria, deficiency of necessary chemicals and bodily malfunctioning. Dealing with these aspects then becomes the major goal of any treatment. On the contrary, Indian patients often subscribe to non-medical causation, such as God's will, karma, spirits and fate for their health problem (Dalal & Misra, 2006). Bodily conditions are considered to be secondary causes of their health problems. This variation in the causal beliefs of doctors and patients lead to a different course of treatment. Joshi (1988) found in his study in Himalayan region that patients seek medical treatment for the secondary (bodily) causes of the problems, whereas for primary causes they visit indigenous healers.

Community Health Workers

In terms of manpower planning, a remarkable achievement was the training of 400,000 of CHW within five years (1977–1982), almost one CHW for each village in the country, constituting the largest health care cadre in the world (Chatterjee, 1993).

These CHWs were trained by medical doctors to take care of common diseases and work as a link between the community and medical staff. This rapid expansion did compromise with the quality in many ways. Nobody knew what kind of training these CHWs should be imparted and very soon these workers began to perceive themselves as village medical practitioners. Later on, the Indian Medical Association opposed this scheme and termed these CHWs as quacks, who were indeed more popular than the medical doctors in many places. In 1981, when the Government of India transferred this scheme to the states, many states which did not commit to this scheme initially started backing out. Lack of availability of state funds made this scheme almost defunct. These workers were rechristened as multipurpose health workers and later, as health guides, but no serious efforts were made to revive the scheme. In fact, this most ambitious scheme of the government lost its direction and relevance.

Under the NRHM, launched by the Union Government in 2005, an effort was made to reconceptualize this scheme as ASHA (Accredited Social Health Activist), recruiting only women health workers. The plan was to identify functionally literate women from the same village and train them for awareness building about health rights. In addition, ASHA is expected to implement national health programmes with the support of local panchayats. This big cadre of more than 400,000 health workers is yet to be effectively inducted in the NRHM scheme. Coming from the same socio-cultural background, these health workers can play an important role in integrating traditional health care systems into national programmes at sub-centre and primary health centres.

Need for Alternative to Western Medicinal System

Modern medicine has not been effective in dealing with a large number of chronic health problems. Many medicines are at the best palliative, life-sustaining with many side effects, causing secondary complications. The horror of long-term use of painkillers and antibiotics has compelled the West to search for the alternative medicines which are effective and safer with less harmful side effects.

Despite opposition from modern medicine, the popularity of alternative medicinal systems is rising worldwide. A study has shown that the use of alternative medicine had risen from 33.8 per cent in 1990 to 42.1 per cent in 1997 (Wetzel, Eisenberg, & Kaptchuk, 1998). The report released by the House of Lords, UK in 2000 suggested that the use of alternative medicine is high and rising. Studies assessing its prevalence in 13 countries concluded that about 31 per cent of cancer patients use some form of complementary and alternative medicine (Cassileth, 1998). In developing nations, where access to modern medicine is severely restricted by the lack of resources and poverty, alternative remedies are quite popular. In Africa, traditional medicine is used for 80 per cent of the primary health care, and in developing nations as a whole more than one-third of the population lack access to modern medicine (WHO, 2005).

A survey of US hospitals by the Health Forum, a subsidiary of the American Hospital Association (2008), found that more than 37 per cent of responding hospitals indicated that they offer one or more alternative medicine therapies, up from 26.5 per cent in 2005. In the United States, increasing numbers of medical colleges have started offering courses in alternative medicine. For example, in three separate research surveys that surveyed 729 schools (125 medical schools offering an MD degree, 25 medical schools offering a Doctor of Osteopathic Medicine degree and 585 schools offering a nursing degree), 60 per cent of the standard medical schools, 95 per cent of osteopathic medical schools and 84.8 per cent of the nursing schools teach some form of alternative medicine (Wetzel et al., 1998). The resurgence of alternative medicine seems to be a worldwide phenomenon.

India's Rich Tradition of Health Care

Ayurveda is the ancient system of medicine in India with a long history of three millenia. It is a comprehensive and holistic system of health care founded on grounded theoretical principles about the physical body and its functioning. Chattopadhyay (1982) argues that Ayurveda is a secular science grounded in observation and experiences, and its therapeutic procedures are empirically testable; religion was superimposition in the later period. Zimmerman (1987) considers Ayurveda a medical science within a modern and broader formulation of the term 'science'. It can be further added in this context that goals of science and spirituality are the same—to help people stay in good health (Vishvanathan, 1997). In Ayurveda, spirit and matter, soul and body, although different, are not alien, insofar as they can be brought together in a healthy relationship with consequences that are mutually beneficial. Its prime concern is not with 'healing' in the narrow sense of curing illness but in the broader sense of promoting health and well-being and prolonging life.

Ayurvedic perspective informs that health is a distributed phenomenon linked with the harmonious operation of a man-environment unit. This inclusive view recognizes the continuity of the body and universe. The continuity of microcosm and macrocosm and sharing in terms of five basic elements (pancha mahābhutas) demands a new approach to health in an inclusive manner (Chattopadhyay, 1982). The interconnectedness and complementarity inherent in nature is the key to unlock the principles of health and well-being. Thus, appropriate conduct (*samyakachara*) can only solve the problem. It includes a regulated lifestyle covering thoughts, actions and food (vichar, achar and ahar).

According to Ayurveda, any disturbance, physical or mental, manifests itself both in the somatic and in the psychic spheres, through the intermediary process of the vitiation of the 'humours'. Ayurvedic therapy aims at correcting the doshas or the imbalances and derangements of the bodily humours (namely, vāta or bodily air, pitta or bile, and kapha or phlegm) and restoring equilibrium. It does so by coordinating all of the material, mental and spiritual resources of the person, recognizing that the essence of these potencies is manifestations of cosmic forces. Medical intervention at the physical level is of four types: diet, activity, purification, and palliation (Svoboda, 1995). In essence, the maintenance of equilibrium is health and, conversely, the disturbance of the equilibrium of tissue elements characterizes the state of disease.

Though Ayurveda is the most prominent and popular alternative system of medicine in India, there are many other indigenous systems which are practised. Some such systems, as mentioned earlier, are Unāni, homeopathy, naturopathy, herbal and so on. These alternative systems of medicine differ from biomedical medicine in many important ways. Alternative medicine greatly relies on the healing powers of nature. It assumes that all of us have the natural ability to heal ourselves. For example, hakims, practising the Unāni system, will, instead of using antibiotics to suppress the infection, would medicate to improve immune system of the patient. Such medication would bolster and allow body's natural healing mechanism to take over. Two, alternative medicines are patient-centred rather than physician or profession-centred. They take into consideration the patient's beliefs and personality in the treatment decision-making. They treat the patient as a person rather than as a body which medical treatment does. Three, alternative medicine generally resorts to the holistic treatment, taking into consideration mental, social and moral conditions of the person. Alternative medicine treats the whole person, not just her/his physical condition. Four, many of these alternative medicines use natural substances, such as herbs, nutritional supplements, botanical plants and so on for the treatment, not synthesized medicines or concentrates. Five, alternative medicines more often deal with prevention and improvement of health, rather than merely on treatment of the diseases. It takes into consideration other factors, such as patient care, diet and anxieties while dealing with the patients. Lastly, alternative medicine practitioner involves family and community in the treatment procedure. Disease is considered to be a social event rather that an individual's pathology. Consequently, family and community are actively engaged in the treatment and healing process.

Challenge of Integrating Diverse Indigenous Systems

To understand the real challenge of integration of diverse indigenous systems of health care, let us briefly review its genesis and efforts made in the past. In 1938, largely as a result of the Freedom Struggle and emphasis on 'swadeshi', the National Planning Committee (NPC) set up by the Indian National Congress took a decision to absorb practitioners of Ayurveda and Unāni systems into the formal health set-up of independent India. In 1946, the Health Ministers' Conference adopted the NPC proposals and resolved to make appropriate financial allocations for:

1. Research, based on the application of scientific methods, in Ayurveda and Unāni;
2. Establishment of colleges and schools for training in diploma degree courses in indigenous systems;

3. Developing postgraduate courses for teaching Indian medicine;
4. Absorption of vaidyas and hakims as doctors, health workers and so on, and
5. Inclusion of departments and practitioners of Indian medicine on national health committees.

As a result of the Conference resolutions, the government set up the Chopra Committee (Ministry of Health, 1948) on the Indigenous Systems of Medicine to work out guidelines for the implementation of the above proposals. The Chopra Committee eventually came out in support of a synthesis of the Indian and Western systems through integrated teaching and research. It recommended that the curriculum be designed to strengthen and supplement one system with the other, with each making up for the other's deficiencies while research should be concentrated on removing useless accretions to Ayurveda and making it intelligible to modern minds since a large portion of the texts were in Sanskrit. The ultimate objective of the research ought to be a synthesis of Indian and Western medicine which was suited to Indian conditions.

The Chopra Committee was followed by the Dave Committee which went into the issue of establishing standards in respect of education and regulation of practice in Indian Systems of Medicine (ISM). The Committee recommended an integrated course of teaching and some states in the Indian Union, in fact, started integrated colleges which taught both modern medicine and Ayurveda. In other states, however, traditional Ayurvedic colleges were also established. Indeed, the political and market forces were not favourable for any integrated approach. The medical practitioners who dominated health care services were not ready to dilute their education and practices to accommodate traditional practices.

As a consequence, the support for integrated medical colleges declined, while pressure for pure Ayurvedic colleges increased. Ayurvedic practitioners and supporters of Ayurveda generally pointed to the popularity of indigenous practitioners, the higher cost of integrated colleges due to the expensive equipment required for teaching Western medicine, the tendency to spend too much time on allopathy, the availability of indigenous graduates for rural practice and finally, the inherent incompatibility of the two systems. Eventually, the supporters of a pure system of education and training for Ayurveda, homeopathy and Unāni system prevailed over the then government. It led to the formation of separate, independent councils for looking after the research, development, training and regulatory aspects of respective ISM. As for research into ISM, the government first set up the Central Council for Research in Indian Medicine and Homeopathy in 1969. The Council guided and supervised research through its five technical advisory boards. This body, however, was dissolved in 1979. In its place, the government decided to set up Central Councils along the lines of the Indian Council for Medical Research.

To promote indigenous systems, the Department of Indian Systems of Medicine and Homoeopathy (ISM&H) was created in 1995. It was renamed as the Department of Ayurveda, Yoga & Naturopathy, Unāni, Siddha and Homoeopathy (AYUSH) in 2003 to provide focused attention to the development of education and research in AYUSH systems. The Department continued to lay emphasis on the upgradation of AYUSH educational standards, quality control and standardization of drugs, improving the availability of medicinal plant material, research and development and awareness generation about the efficacy of the systems domestically and internationally. The draft of National Health Policy Document (2015) has put greater emphasis on promoting AYUSH and allocating greater funding for indigenous systems.

However, if we look in terms of funding support, ISM always got ridiculously low funding out of the total health allocation. In the First Five Year Plan (1952–1957), the allocation for ISM was about 1 per cent of the total health budget; it increased marginally in subsequent plans but came down to 1.3 per cent in the Seventh Plan (1985–1990). The total allocation was raised from ₹35 crores to ₹100 crores in the year 2004, and this announcement drew applause from the starved ISM sector. It is appropriate to mention here that the total allocation for the Ministry of Health the same year was ₹4,319 crores and ISM got a mere 2.5 per cent of the whole budget. This allocation was increased steeply, to more than ₹1,000 crores in the annual budget of the Union Government in 2013, which was still mere 3.3 per cent of the total health budget. Banerjee's (2004) observation that the Indian systems of medicine continued to be marginalized and have a limited role public health care system holds even after a decade.

Apart from their traditional practice, AYUSH practitioners are now permitted to prescribe allopathic medicines in some cases. They are also allowed to terminate unwanted pregnancies within the rules.

Medical fraternity has opposed to such permission to traditional practitioners for the fear of possible abuse. The government has no policy to regulate and integrate indigenous systems within the health care programme, which is dominated by medical doctors. The worst victims of this official apathy towards indigenous systems are the rural poor who otherwise have no access to modern medicine.

Folk Healing as the Third Alternative

As discussed in the preceding chapter, folk (or faith) healing coexists in India along with modern medicine and traditional medicinal systems. These healing practices are often labelled as magico-religious, which are alleged to be practised by primitive and uneducated people. At the best, their efficacy is considered to be merely a placebo effect. In India, faith healers are found in every corner of the country, comprising shamans, mystics, tantrics, priests, ojhas, yogis, gurus, babas and others. Though these healing practices are consistent with the cultural beliefs and have popular mass support, these are seen with scepticism by most of the government agencies and scientific community. However, as mentioned in the previous chapter, the popularity of such folk (or faith) healing practices has not declined in the present times, rather such healing places are getting more crowded. Their diversity and local variants constituted a rich tapestry of health care practices in India. It may be noted that most of these folk-healing practices and associated systems have evolved in the long history, have been practised for thousands of years and are time-tested and culturally compatible (Dalal, 2013; Dalal & Ray, 2005). These practices survived primarily on popular support and being integral to community life. The WHO estimated that in many countries, 80 per cent or more of the population living in rural areas are catered by traditional practitioners and birth attendants (Bodeker, 2004). Folk healing along with other systems of medicine provides a whole range of health services to cater to physical, mental, social and spiritual health of local communities.

It is impossible to have a precise count of the number of these folk healers, but according to a rough assessment, their number may cross one million mark (*Times of India*, 15 July 2013). If we add this figure to 650,000 medical practitioners and 686,000 traditional practitioners,

India has one of the best patient-practitioner-ratio in the world. India's health policies need to be properly formulated to judiciously utilize all three systems of health and healing to meet health needs of the masses.

Weaving Together Different Systems of Health Care

In 1973, David Werner's book *Where There Is No Doctor* was published in Spanish and an English edition was brought out in 1977. The book is a practical guide for those who work in the rural areas or in the areas where no medical doctor is available. It is considered a complete health care guide which successfully combines modern concepts of public health care with locally available resources and know-how. The book became an instant success all over the world, a must book for all those who work in the non-Western rural region. The WHO, UNICEF and World Bank promoted this book, and recommended it for all those who work in the developing world. After Bible, it is the most sold book in the world which is translated into 46 languages and its English edition is into the thirteenth edition. Working within the Western medicinal system, the book is a good example of utilizing local know-how in providing first-level medical services. This health guide is not a substitute for medical doctors, but is for paramedical staff until specialized medical care is available.

It should be borne in mind that the integration of these diverse systems of medicine is not an easy task. People in India have been using these multiple systems for centuries and have a fair understanding as to how they work. All forms of medicine, from faith healing to home remedies to Ayurvedic prescriptions thrived on popular support, though competition and rivalry among different systems were also there. The dominance of Western medicine over all indigenous systems in the present time has changed the scenario radically. Labelled as primitive, unscientific and superstitious, many of these indigenous healing systems are struggling for their survival. The other argument is that in the face of mounting evidences of the failure of Western medicine, a revival of indigenous systems is in the offing. For an average Indian with rising cost of medicine and diagnostic procedures, medical treatment is getting out of bounds and indigenous treatment is the only option. This makes it all the more important to discuss the possibilities of bringing Western and indigenous medicine into the fold of primary health services to reach out to a larger section of the society.

Indigenous practices are holistic in nature and faith in them keeps patients' hopes alive even under adverse circumstances. These medicines intend to deal with the mind and emotional state of the physically sick person and help in creating a psychological environment necessary for any recovery to be enduring. The efficacy of indigenous therapies is widely acknowledged and there is mounting empirical evidence that many of these work, even if we do not comprehend how and why?

The important question is how to integrate indigenous healing practices with modern medicine? There are two schools of thoughts in this regard. The first school views indigenous systems as based on fundamentally different assumptions about human life, health and illness, which, in no way, can reconcile with the theories of biomedicine. The indigenous medicines attempt to restore the balance of mind–body–soul and treat patients holistically. The medical approach, on the contrary, treats a patient as a passive organism and focuses only on bodily aspects of the health problem. These fundamental differences in these two approaches are reflected in the differences in the formulation of the theories pertaining to the causation of diseases, pharmacology and drug action, dietetics and nutrition, diagnostics and so on (Shankar, 1992). Thus, those who subscribe to the first school consider Western and indigenous medicines irreconcilable and prefer them being practised rather independently.

Many critiques of this school consider indigenous healing practices as unscientific and of very limited efficacy. The sceptics of alternative practices argue that the symptomatic relief to an, otherwise, ineffective therapy can be attributed to the placebo effect or to the natural recovery from or the cyclical nature of an illness or to the possibility that the person never originally had a real illness. However, studies show that mainstream medications may also show the placebo effect. An analysis of the six most widely prescribed antidepressants submitted to the US Food and Drug Administration showed that approximately 80 per cent of the response to medication was duplicated in placebo control groups and improvement at the highest doses of medication was not different from improvement at the lowest doses (as reported in Papakostas & Christodoulou, 2010). In fact, many of these alternative medicines are found to have a transformational experience that changed their world view, relationship and self-concept, and identify the remedy with commitment to a social cause and personal growth.

The second school of thoughts though acknowledges differences in the two treatment approaches, sees many possibilities of developing a unified health care delivery system. Its emphasis is on a creative synthesis between these two systems to develop a new Indian model of health care. The vast local resources of indigenous healers need to be mobilized to bolster the crumbling public health services where different medicinal systems can work under one roof. There are many possibilities and we need to learn from the experiences and experiments going on in the field.

India's rich health care traditions and well-developed indigenous practices have not been seriously incorporated in the health planning. The public health care programmes need to be more responsive to aspirations and practices of the common people. Apart from providing curative services, rural health centres should also be the nucleus of all-round socio-economic-spiritual development. To achieve this dream, it is important that social workers, school teachers, religious leaders and even faith healers are closely associated with the activities of the health centres. Indonesian health services have shown the way, where indigenous healers are trained to refer serious cases to medical professionals, but these patients come back to the indigenous healer for holy water, once they are cured (Sinha, 1990). Such practices not only relieve pressure on the medical practitioners but also take care of both curing and healing aspects of the disease.

Plural health care practices have always been India's strength. The Ayurvedic practitioners, tantrics, yoga teachers, priests, hakims and God-men have always offered a range of services, sometimes complementing each other, other times working independently. It was for the patients and their families to decide whose services they would seek. The indigenous health practitioners had thrived not on official patronage but on public support and faith. The same thing cannot be said about modern medicine which is promoted by the government, even at the cost of indigenous systems. This scenario is changing now in the last two–three decades as more and more people all over the world are seeking indigenous medicines for the ailments modern medicine has no treatment for. Indian indigenous medicines have much to offer to alleviate human pain and suffering.

Sri Lanka has the health care practice which is a good example of possible integration at the level of service delivery. There, all systems are allowed to practice freely but an enquiry is mandatory if there is any casualty of suspicious nature. This enquiry is conducted by a group of respectable local people. Because of this mandatory requirement, many indigenous practitioners refer serious cases to medical doctors. Such formal collaboration between modern and traditional medical sectors can grow to meet all health eventualities. Sri Lanka has a very developed legislative and policy frameworks for the promotion and development of traditional medicine. It has a separate Ministry of Ayurveda for the last four decades, something which India did much later. Sri Lanka, with its meagre resources, has evolved one of the best health care systems in Asia and has achieved health targets almost on par with the Western standards.

The new health care system needs to be made more broad-based so that it can handle all the facets of the problem, including public education about health and hygiene. Apart from providing curative services, rural health centres should have been the nucleus of all-round development. To achieve this dream, it is important that social workers, school teachers, religious leaders and even faith healers are closely associated with the activities of the health centres. Indonesian health services have also shown the way to integrate traditional healers in health care services. Such integration of diverse systems not only provides more options to the general public but also takes care of both curing and healing aspects of the recovery from a disease. It also relieves pressure on the medical practitioners.

The pragmatism of Indian patients, in the light of culturally and religiously diverse medical systems, helps them choose the best mode of treatment under the circumstances. At the same time, context-sensitive Indian medical practitioners learn from their clinical experience to complement their diverse medical practices. Cultural sensibilities and practical considerations have substantially shaped the practice of modern medicine and medical technology in India over a century. Modern medicine in India has thus influenced and has been influenced by Ayurvedic and other medical systems of India (Khare, 1996). This alignment of traditional and modern medicine is occurring more or less spontaneously. A large number of modern Indian physicians and surgeons prescribe Ayurvedic medicines, often in combination with modern drugs. Most Ayurvedic medicines are known to have few or no harmful effects. Traditional practitioners also routinely prescribe modern medicine for quick results. This trend is, of course, not uniform and fraught with problems.

The challenge of providing health services to over 1.25 billion Indians is indeed very unnerving. About three-quarter of this population is under the poverty line and cannot afford expensive medical treatment. The problem is acuter in the case of those who reside in villages and remote areas. They need inexpensive treatment for common ailments which is locally available. This is the area where different systems of medicine can work in unison. A modest beginning of providing basic medical aid can be made by utilizing the vast cadre of community health workers (CHWs or ASHA workers). These health workers can be an important link between various schools of health care providers. The CHWs can be suitably trained to map and utilize local health resources. If the local faith healers who are respected and trusted by the villagers can be identified and trained in holistic health practices, it can provide the first-level services. He/she may assist the village panchayat in meeting the basic health needs and act as a link between the health agencies and local people. In addition, there should be a massive effort in health education in the entire country, through school teachers, panchayat members, youth clubs, Mahila Mandals and community development workers to help people inculcate a more rational and scientific understanding of both traditional and modern medicine. In this, vast national networks of voluntary organizations can also play an important role.

While discussing the possibilities of integration of ISM at the level of primary health care, we need to be wary of some new trends emerging in the global market. The market requirement of standardization, commercialization and pharmaceuticalization of the medicine has substantially changing profile and practices of the ISM in the arena of health. There is an apparent paradox. While these processes have conferred a new legitimacy on traditional systems, their radical transformation has meant that even as their face value has appreciated their innate potential as systems of healing have declined. Indigenous medicine is in danger of falling prey to pharmaceuticalization, that is, using the pharmacology of these systems to create new pharmaceuticals, or medicinal commodities, that could be sold independently of the original line of treatment (Nandy & Visvanathan, 1990). Such commodification of indigenous systems may give a false impression that its popularity is on increase, but in essence, it could be allopathization of the Indian systems. Thus, while getting integrated into the primary health care, it is equally important that Indian systems of medicine preserve their humanistic–holistic character, and not swayed away by market forces.

5

Participatory Rehabilitation of Poor with Disability

In a developing country, like India, the challenge of rehabilitation and improving the quality of life of people with disabilities is to be viewed from historical, cultural and socio-economic perspectives. The rehabilitation practices of a society cannot be understood without making sense of its cultural beliefs, social practices and crisis management strategies. As Groce (1990) argued, societies develop their characteristic patterns of coping with physical disability, depending on the way disability is understood and the resources to cope with it are identified. Historical events, sacred texts, social institutions and so on, all contribute in understanding the disablement and its implications. In this endeavour, it is imperative that culture and traditions are viewed as strengths rather than impediments in improving the quality of life of people with disability. These cultural factors coupled with the socio-economic status of the people with disability play an important role in determining the efficacy of developmental schemes and programmes intended for people with disabilities. This chapter examines the perception of disability in India and its implications for the rehabilitation of poor with disability. It also examines how prevalent disability attitudes lead to discrimination and exclusion from social mainstream. The chapter deliberates over the development programmes which are likely to succeed in the rehabilitation of poor with disability.

Indian has always remained a pluralistic society with multiple traditions weaving a multicoloured pattern, contributed by the waves of immigrants with different faiths and cultures, in the long history. It is important to note that these are living traditions with a history of dissents, protests and reforms and efforts to adapt to the new realities. In the resulting diversity, two institutions, which were common to all traditions and which survived many crises, are family and religion. These were the decisive factors that played a role in shaping the rehabilitation practices within Indian society. Family, as a basic social unit played its crucial role in uniting and supporting its members and giving them a social identity. Like family, religion also pervaded all spheres of life, as a major force behind all social decisions and activities. This scenario has not changed much in spite of all global, economic and technological changes affecting the local communities. Understanding the socio-economic background of these families, their social and religious practices, is essential for the success of any rehabilitation programme at the grassroots level.

In recent times, rehabilitation policies and programmes are increasingly emphasizing participatory models. These participatory models envisage an active role for local communities in planning and implementing rehabilitation schemes. Unless there is knowledge and understanding of the native culture, no community-based scheme can succeed in mobilizing local participation. Any discussion on local culture can thus have three objectives. First is to ensure better understanding of needs, aspirations and expectations of the local communities; second is to plan better rehabilitation programmes and their implementation with community support, including people with disabilities and their families; and third is to identify indigenous knowledge and resources and utilize it in achieving the goals of rehabilitation to improve the life conditions of people with disabilities and their families.

In the next section, religious beliefs and family practices will be closely examined for their salience in forming traditional attitudes towards physical disability in India and its implications for rehabilitation of the poor with the disability. Some recent research studies in this area are also discussed.

The Concept of Divine Retribution

Indians, in general, have an ambivalent attitude towards people with disability. In dealing with someone with a disability, people are caught in an avoid- help kind of a conflicting situation and feel anxious in their presence. The religious beliefs about disability only add to this confusion. There is a belief in divine punishment in all religions and people tend to accept the condition of disablement as something they deserved. This punishment is presumed to be meted out for their sinful acts, and one can overcome the resultant suffering by engaging in morally right behaviour. The other prevalent notion is that God inflicts suffering on good people to test their resilience and inner strength. In either case, one is expected to respect God's will. Those people who are more fortunate are exhorted by religious texts to show pity and compassion to all those who are suffering. *Manusmriti*, the ancient charter of social conduct, impelled people to spare a part of their material resources for their hapless fellow-beings, to support their daily living (Prabhu, 1963). The Dharmashastra called upon all householders to look after the weak and disabled, and those who did so were ensured a place in heaven (Kuppuswamy, 1977).

Hindu scriptures have provided elaborate commentaries on 'why do people suffer?' The theory of karma is propounded to explain all kinds of suffering. This theory implies that if one has committed misdeeds in previous births, one has to inevitably bear the consequences. Disability is held to be a punishment for the sins of previous births and one is called upon to accept it as divine retribution. This notion of a just world is firmly ingrained in the Hindu mind and is frequently invoked to explain whatever happens in one's life (Paranjpe, 1984; Radhakrishnan, 1926). Belief in the theory of karma has very often led to a ready acceptance of physical disability, with little effort in the direction of improving life conditions of such people. It is presumed to be a deterrent to collective efforts put in by persons with disabilities to assert their right of equal access to social opportunities.

So strong was the belief in the theory of karma as a potent cause of all human suffering throughout the ages that people with disability were never identified as a separate group, nor were they segregated on this count. In most of the earlier literature (Prabhu, 1963), destitute, widows, aged, diseased and disabled people were put together in one category, under one roof. The shelter homes built by benevolent kings and nobles were for the benefit of all those who had no other place to go, whether their problem was social, economic or physical. This practice continued all through the medieval and colonial period. So much so, that even in the constitution of free India, they were bracketed together. Article 41 of the Indian Constitution adopted in 1950 reads, "the State shall, within the limits of its economic capacity and development, make effective provisions for securing the right to work, to education, and to public assistance in cases of unemployment, old age, sickness and disablement."

Studies conducted by the author and his colleagues have clearly shown that people frequently attribute their disease and disability to metaphysical factors, particularly to their own karma. Dalal (2015) studied causal beliefs of hospital patients who were under treatment for a wide range of physical diseases—coronary heart disease, tuberculosis, cancer and orthopaedic problems. These patients consistently attributed their physical problems to their own karma. In general, causal attribution to metaphysical factors (God's will, fate and karma) was consistently high. These patients, however, did not attribute their recovery to their karma, as much as to the doctor, God and other factors. It is to be mentioned here that most of these patients were rural, uneducated and from poor families. Similar findings were obtained in the case of physical disability also. In a study conducted in rural areas, Dalal (2000b) found that people with disabilities, their families as well as the community members often attribute physical disability to the cosmic factors—fate, God's will and karma. Religious beliefs thus seem to be providing important explanations for both diseases and disabilities.

Such causal profile may lead to the erroneous conclusion that these people are irrational, passive, fatalistic and 'otherworldly'. When one attempts to view the situation as an insider, the pertinent question would not be one of fatalism but would relate to the structure of opportunities. Poverty, lack of medical facilities, poor hygiene and unsupportive government machinery puts them in a predicament where their own efforts prove repeatedly futile. Also, when the existing body of knowledge and technology fails to provide solace and the outcome of their efforts are negative, people learn to accept the outcomes in a spirit of resignation (Dube, 1990). When fresh opportunities did surface, or when new technical choices were available, the same people did not lack initiative in trying them out. Joshi (1988), in a study of tribes in the foothills of the Himalayas, observed that people are pragmatic in their causal attributions. When they see a medical doctor for their sickness, they talk about the organic symptoms, but the same people while visiting a traditional healer articulate their sickness in terms of metaphysical causality—God's wrath, spirits and so on. The patients intuitively learn to keep these two aspects of the disease separate. Kleinman (1988) in his extensive work in China, India and other Asian countries found that in all these places, traditional healing and biomedical treatment coexist and are not perceived as contradictory.

This all-pervasive faith in supernatural powers as potent causes and remedies for disabling diseases has led to the proliferation of healing centres in the country. These healing centres have retained their popularity throughout the ages and are visited by a large population. Cutting across all cross sections, people believe in the healing powers of these shrines and frequent them regularly in the hope of a miracle.

Disability and Poverty

Apart from cultural beliefs, another factor is the socio-economic status of the people with disabilities. According to the United Kingdom Department for International Development (Yeo, 2005), 10,000 individuals with disabilities die each day as a result of extreme poverty, showing that the connection between these two constructs is especially problematic. Heumann (2012) referring to the link between disability and development indicated that of the 650 million people living with disabilities today 80 per cent of them live in developing countries. In most of the developing countries like India, disability and poverty are inseparable. They tend to go hand in hand, forming a cycle of cumulative causation (Acton, 1983). Disabled people are more likely to be poor than their non-disabled peers, and people living in poverty are more likely to become disabled than those who are not (Elwan, 1999). Most international aid agencies and scholars agree that poverty and disability are causally intertwined. This essay primarily focuses on rehabilitation and well-being of the poor with disabilities in India and on the development programmes initiated by the government and other agencies.

Many government departments, survey organizations, international aid agencies and national NGOs have conducted surveys in recent years to provide a comprehensive picture of disablement. Many of these surveys have come to an estimation that people with disabilities make up approximately 10 per cent of any country's population, and that people with disabilities represent over 20 per cent of the world's poor (World Bank, 2005). Stated differently, three out of four disabled people belong to the poorest strata of the society. Worse, more than 50 per cent of preventable disabilities are directly linked to poverty. According to Javed Abidi (2004) of the National Centre for Promotion of Employment for Disabled People (NCPEDP), as many as 70 per cent of the disabled people of India reside in rural areas and 50 per cent of them are extremely poor. A report by the state-run National Commission for Enterprises in the Unorganized Sector (NCEUS, 2007) found that 77 per cent of Indians, that is, 836 million people, lived on less than 20 rupees per day, with most of them working in informal labour sector with no job or social security, living in abject poverty. The World Bank Report (2008) entitled *People with Disabilities in India: From Commitments to Outcomes* noted that the disabled people are subject to multiple deprivations and they are the most excluded from education. The report observed that children with disability are around four to five times less likely to go to school than the children from scheduled tribes and scheduled castes. The International Labour Organization (ILO) (2003) report shows that only 20 per cent of the people with disabilities have some meaningful employment, the statistics presumably include self-employment and underemployment.

The poor with disability are caught in the complex web of causal factors. Bodily (including physical, neural and cognitive) impairment imposes various capacity restrictions on an individual which are further aggravated by a combination of social, psychological, environmental and policy impediments, resulting in disability. Bodily impairment is thus not a necessary condition for making someone disabled. Disability arises from the interaction of functional aspects of the person's impairments and health incapacities, and the physical and psychosocial environment they live in. Some of the psychosocial factors responsible for one's disability are social and economic discrimination, inaccessible physical environment, socially segregating and counter-productive disability institutions and policies, low expectations, low self-image and self-reinforcing exclusion and special health and rehabilitation needs. This listing could be endless and typically constitute the life conditions of people with disabilities. When these factors are compounded by limiting access to health care, adequate nutrition, poor hygiene, health and inaccessible educational and employment opportunities and economic impoverishment, people are caught in an endemic cycle of disability–poverty. According to a study (Lee, 1999), poor nutrition and sanitation alone are estimated to cause impairments in over 100 million people worldwide. Poverty may lead to delayed evaluation by a physician and, therefore, may cause disability. This disability may exclude people socially and economically, which makes them poorer and gives them even less access to care, which in turn may aggravate their disability (Birbeck, 2000). A study done in Cambodia shows that poor people lack access to basic health care which means that simple infections, illnesses and injuries could result in permanent disability because they go untreated or are mistreated (as reported in Elwan, 1999). All informants who became disabled later in life indicated that they became poorer after they were disabled, and most said they had become much poorer. This might be explained by the fact that disability can have an impact on a person's ability to work and earn a living (Thomas, 2005a). Poverty also appears to be a high-risk factor for unintentional injuries, resulting in disability. Consequently, people with disability, irrespective of their other advantages, are more likely to live in poverty.

Mitigating the negative consequences of the two-way relationship between disability and poverty is increasingly recognized to be a necessary component of any disability rehabilitation programme. No poverty programme can be effective if it ignores its poorest minority, and no disability programme will be successful if it ignores the conditions faced by most disabled people. According to the World Bank (2005), failure to account for this differential by development programmes and strategies "can seriously limit the effectiveness of programmes designed to promote economic and social well-being."

The contention of this chapter is that challenge of disability–poverty is not just that of economic development, which is the main thrust of government policies and aid agencies. This simplistic approach has neither yielded tangible outcomes nor made any dent in the massive task of disability rehabilitation in India and in other developing countries. This review chapter attempts to critically examine some salient psychosocial factors which explain the downward nature of the disability–poverty spiral, such as social exclusion, negative and discriminatory attitude, employment impediments and accessibility. The chapter has also highlighted some of the psychosocial barriers that impede any meaningful participation of local communities in the rehabilitation process. Understanding and breaking these psychosocial and also physical barriers to participation are the only way to facilitate upward mobility of the poor with disability and improve their quality of life.

In the later part of this chapter, a schematic model depicting the interlinkages among these factors is also proposed. The chapter also explores the possibility of changing the direction of the disability–poverty spiral to improve the quality of life of people with disabilities.

Poor Quality of Disability Statistics

Disability statistics are notoriously unreliable; at best, they only provide a crude estimation of the existing scenario. The wide variation in the nature and severity of disabilities makes them less amenable to quantification and statistical analysis. Even the same disability has different implications and consequences for different stakeholders. Often the import of these disabilities is highly context-specific and the important question may be 'who' has the disability rather than 'what' disability one has. The situation is further compounded by the fact that disabilities are hard to define, their definitions and meaning keep changing in different societies and cultures. It is despite the fact that WHO (2001) has developed a universal classification system International Classification of Functioning Disability and Health (ICF). This classification system is based on the Western conception of disability and often not practical in the developing countries. There are no reliable measuring instruments. Disability survey data tend to be unsuitable for cross-survey comparison because the sizes of disability populations and the severities of disabilities recorded depend on underlying social and environmental contexts. Elwan (1999) has found that differences in disability definitions, information collection methodologies and capacities for diagnosis cause significant variations and inaccuracies. In her extensive review of the disability research, Ghai (2010) has noted that within the documented research in India, there does not seem to be any uniform terminology which the researchers have used in disability area.

Disability is also inherently difficult to observe, as cultural issues like stigma and prejudice adversely affect obtaining reliable and authentic data from disability surveys and statistics. Disabled people are often described as invisible in sociological studies (Harriss-White, 1996) because households often restrict the participation of their disabled family members in community activities and often fail to reveal disabled family members to surveyors (Thomas, 2005b; Yeo & Moore, 2003).

It is difficult to map the extent and severity of physical disability due to lack of any effective system of medical assessment and rehabilitation services. It is ironical that rehabilitation services in India are primarily based on the medical model though, in reality, these services hardly reach to more than 2 per cent of the population with disability. In the absence of any local and referral services, it is impossible to have any realistic appraisal of the prevalent disability. In the year 2007, there were over 550,000 registered medical doctors and over 700,000 registered non-allopathic (non-Western) doctors in India. There is no actual count of rehabilitation specialists, other paramedical personnel and traditional practitioners working in the field. With a vast pool of formerly trained and traditional practitioners, the health and rehabilitation services still elude the poor and disabled who need them the most. In the absence of any credible database, it is difficult to fix accountability on one hand and assess the outcome of any development programme aiming to improve the life conditions of poor with disabilities on the other. This situation is common to all developing countries.

WHO Definition of Disability

In 1980, the WHO developed a three-dimensional framework to define disability. According to this framework, these three dimensions are impairment, disability and handicap. According to WHO (1980), 'impairment' refers to any loss or abnormality of psychological, physiological or anatomical structure or function. It is characterized by losses or abnormalities that may be temporary or permanent. It includes the existence of an anomaly, defect or loss of a limb, organ or tissue, or other structures of the body. 'Disability' implies any restriction or lack (resulting from impairment) of ability to perform an activity in the manner or within the range considered normal for a human being. It entails deficiencies of specific activity, performance and behaviour. These could be of temporary or permanent, reversible or irreversible, progressive or regressive nature. Disability may arise as a result of physical or sensory impairments. 'Handicap' denotes a disadvantage for an individual, resulting from an impairment that limits or prevent the fulfilment of a role that is normal (depending on age, sex and social and cultural factors) for an individual. It is characterized by a misfit between individual's performance and status in accordance with the expected behaviour.

In brief, impairment means any loss or abnormality of organic nature, disability refers to the lack of ability to perform in a normal range and handicap refers to a disadvantage (cultural, social, economic and environmental) resulting from the impairment or disability. Clearly, handicap is not an inevitable consequence of the disability. It is dependent on interactions between a whole range of social, cultural and behavioural variables. Thus, whereas impairment and disability suggest disturbances at the individual level, handicap refers to medical as well as psycho-social-cultural aspects, involving family, community and professionals.

Many practitioners and experts in the field of disability pointed out many limitations of the WHO definition of disability. First, there is a good deal of overlap between impairment, disability and handicap, the way these are defined. Second, disability cannot be an all or none condition but can be a matter of degree. Third, handicap largely depends on social, cultural, ecological and political conditions of a region and no international standards can be fixed in such cases. For greater clarity and planning of rehabilitation programmes, the need was felt to modify the WHO definition.

After much deliberation for years, the WHO (2001) reformulated earlier three-dimensional model of disability in terms of human functioning—impairment, activity limitations and participation restriction. Impairments are problems in the functioning of the body—it could be some loss of functioning or malfunctioning at physical, neural or cognitive level. Activity limitations are problems in the capacity to perform activities, sensory or mental, simple or complex. And finally, participation restrictions are environmentally imposed limitations of a person across a range of personal, professional and social activities. These three dimensions of disability arise from an interaction between the health condition of an individual and his or her physical, social and attitudinal environment.

The WHO model of disability posits that impairment is intrinsic to the person, but participation restriction is determined mostly by the social and physical environment. It identifies these socio-psychological and physical barriers which severely restrict the participation of poor people with disability in social and economic activities. It also highlights the complex ways in which these barriers result in undesired consequences in terms of education and unemployment status for keeping them as the poorest among the poor.

Attitudinal Barriers

Disability is often in the mind of the perceiver (Wright, 1983). Disability policies, programmes and practices of any country are manifestations of attitudes that people in different cultures share. It is, therefore, easy to assume that in developing countries where basic life conditions are hard to maintain, such prejudices would have far more dehumanizing consequences. People in their struggle to survive and feed their dependents go through all kinds of exploitations and self-degrading experiences. There is poverty, illness, illiteracy and massive unemployment, leading to severe competition for diminishing resources. Under such conditions, persons with disabilities are one of the most vulnerable groups, which suffer more due to societal prejudices than due to their disabling physical condition (Dalal, 2006; Ghai, 2001).

Attitudes are generally understood in terms of their three components—cognitive, affective and behavioural. In the context of disability attitudes, these three components have specific meanings. A cognitive component of the positive attitude towards persons with disability would refer to a belief that these people can be productive members of the community, that these people can and should decide what is good for them and that it is possible for them to lead a normal life. At the affective level, the positive attitude would refer to feeling and liking and their acceptance as members of one's own group. At the behavioural level, positive attitude implies creating conditions which can facilitate their efforts towards the goal of self-reliance and towards socio-economic development of the entire community (Dalal & Pande, 1995). It seems that the negative attitude is one of the major reasons why people are generally apathetic and show low motivation to get involved in disability rehabilitation programmes. Social and psychological theories have convincingly argued that the way people behave is largely dictated by the attitudes and beliefs they hold (e.g., Ajzen & Fishbein, 1980). The three-component model of disability attitudes is useful, not only in understanding the nature of such attitudes but also in understanding the basis of many prejudices. These three components are interrelated, yet they serve as distinct predictors of the way people relate to the persons with disability. For example, the affective component could be a better predictor of a personal bond with friends and family members whereas evaluative component could be a better predictor of negative or positive comparison of 'poor and disabled' with other ethnic groups (Esses & Beaufoy, 1994). The negative attitudes people hold about disability persist in the developing countries. Berman, Dalal and Anthony (1984) found in their study that the overall attitude people hold towards the disabled is that of a patronizing nature. Mallory (1993) observed that in developing countries, traditional attitudes of pity and charity are changing rather marginally. Such attitudes have far-reaching consequences for persons with disabilities. As the ESCAP Report (1993, p. 5) states in the context of Asian and Pacific region,

> This is largely because negative social attitudes exclude persons with disabilities from an equal share in their entitlements as citizens. Negative attitudes also curtail the opportunities of people with disabilities, resulting in having less social contacts and close personal relationships with others.

Miles (1996), on the basis of his study in Pakistan and also studies carried out in 30 other countries, noted that the progressive development is from negative, stigmatizing and rejecting attitudes, through pity and compassion towards willingness to accept the physically challenged persons on equal terms. Studies have shown that females tend to have a more positive attitude than males towards the disabled and the younger generation has a more positive attitude than the older generation (Bakheit & Shanmugalingam, 1997). Regarding employment, the World Bank Report (2008) shows that the assessment of people with disabilities for their capability to succeed on the job is low. Surprisingly, these assessments are also shared by people with disabilities. However, any such general conclusion needs to be tested with some standardized measures of attitudes and beliefs.

The idea that symptoms of poverty promote prejudice finds support in Gunnar Myrdal's *An American Dilemma* (1944), which presents an analysis of the causal connections between poverty and prejudice experienced by the Afro-American population in the United States. The cumulative causation described by Myrdal mirrors the relationship between the poverty of people with disabilities and the social stigmatization they face. The greater the prejudice towards disabled people, the fewer the opportunities they have to earn a living, and the poorer and more destitute they become, thus reinforcing the prejudice and stigmatization. Negative attitudes are expressed in different ways—sometimes subtly, sometimes bluntly and sometimes viciously. People who find it socially undesirable to express such attitudes publicly invent their own indirect ways of expressing them. Sometimes such attitudes are camouflaged and it takes a while to identify them.

Much of the research on poor people has linked poverty with social, psychological and cultural aspects to explain why people are poor in the society. In a now famous study, Feagin (1972) interviewed 1,017 Americans and asked them about their explanations of poverty. He categorized their responses as individualistic (blaming poverty on dispositional factors within poor people), fatalistic (blaming poverty on fate or bad luck) or structural (blaming poverty on society). He reported that 53 per cent of his respondents gave high importance to individualistic items, 22 per cent to structural factors and 18 per cent to fatalistic factors. Feather (1974) conducted a similar study in Australia. Many such studies conducted in the 1980s in India have also tried to suggest that poor and underprivileged groups have cognitive, motivational and intellectual deficits (see Mohanty & Misra, 2000 for a review). These studies have shown that the poor as compared to the non-poor, lack qualities, disposition, skill, motivation and values necessary for socio-economic development. The emphasis is on studying poor as 'individuals', ignoring their socio-cultural background in justifying poverty of the 'poor'. This blaming of the victim was the basis for many social intervention studies conducted in the 1970s and 1980s in India. It was only in a later period that a need to broaden the conceptual framework of poverty research was felt, and contextual and process factors were taken into consideration with an aim to alleviate the poverty.

Attitudes create further disablement for poor people with disabilities, adding to their deprivation and daunting life conditions. Negative attitudes become formidable barriers in their struggle to survive and sustain on any meagre means of livelihood they have. The detrimental effects of negative attitudes are compounded if we view these attitudes in the larger perspective. One is the spread effect. Often, at times, negative evaluation of the condition of disability spreads to influence the evaluation of other non-impaired characteristics. Such spread effect, the power of single characteristic to evoke inferences about a person, was demonstrated in many studies (Hewstone, 1994). These studies evidenced that the term 'disability' or 'poor' can evoke responses about various presumed dispositions of such a person. These responses are not casual; they indicate the respondent's generalized and stereotyped views about the target person or group. People generalize from physical or economic attributes to affective and behavioural characteristics. Such stereotypes, once formed, are resistant to change and form the justification for all kinds of prejudices and discrimination. Two such attitudes and beliefs are often internalized by the poor with disabilities to conform to social expectations. They accept their lot and also the justification offered by others. The Disability-Attitude-Belief-Behaviour (DABB) study (Dalal, Pande, Dhawan, Dwijendra & Berry, 2000) has shown that people with disability internalize negative attitudes about themselves and do not endeavour to improve their lot. Those with disabilities often go through conflicting mental states, where on one hand, they align with the perpetrators who exploit and harm them and on the other, they resent the same group for frustrating their aspiration to access existing resources.

Factors such as prejudice and discrimination are more serious impediments in the fight against poverty and disability than the so-called economic factors. Media and public awareness can play a salutary role in making state and social institutions more responsive to the needs of the disabled and in reducing poverty. Working towards social equity for people with disabilities and changing society's attitudes towards disability can act as catalysts to bring people out of the vicious poverty–disability cycle.

Stigma and Discrimination

The concept of stigma became a popular area of research in social sciences after the pioneering work of Goffman (1963). Referring to stigma as 'spoiled identity', Goffman focused on micro-social processes within which the self is created and maintained. Goffman applied the term (negative) stigma to any condition, attribute, trait or behaviour that symbolically marked off the bearer as 'culturally unacceptable' or inferior, with consequent feelings of shame, guilt and disgrace. He distinguished between three types of stigma. These are associated with the body, individual character and group membership. Along the same lines, Stafford and Scott (1986, pp. 80, 81) defined stigma as "a characteristic of persons that is contrary to a norm of a social unit" where, a 'norm' is defined as a "shared belief that a person ought to behave in a certain way at a certain time." Crocker and others (1993, p. 505) suggest that "stigmatised individuals possess (or are believed to possess) some attribute, or characteristic, that conveys a social identity that is devalued in a particular social context."

The stigma thus refers to some attribute 'within the person' rather than a label that others affix to the person. Consider how the term 'stigma' directs our attention differently than a term like 'discrimination'. Whereas 'discrimination' focuses attention on people or on the agency that purports rejection and exclusion—those who do the discrimination—'stigma' directs attention to the people who are the recipients of these behaviours (Sayce, 1998). Thus, the terms we use may lead to "different understandings of where responsibility lies for the 'problem'" and consequently to "different prescriptions for action" (Sayce, 1998). Negative attitude and prejudice build up justification for stigmatizing a person or a group.

Disability in this context is not simply a physical condition but an ontology—a condition of one's being. Stigma, in that case, is not a by-product of disability, but its very substance. On the level of social relationships, the disabled person presents a counterpoint to normality. Consistent with this view, Fine and Asch (1988) enumerated five assumptions that form the basis for stigmatizing people with disability. These assumptions are (a) that disability is located solely in biology, (b) the problems of the disabled are due to disability-produced impairment, (c) the disabled person is a 'victim', (d) disability is central to the disabled person's self-concept, self-definition, social comparisons and reference groups and (e) having a disability is synonymous with needing help and social support.

Stigma and discrimination exist in a vicious circle. Stigma allows or encourages discriminatory attitudes. These attitudes are often reflected in discriminatory behaviour that results in acts of discrimination. Acts of discrimination draw attention to or increase stigma. Discrimination can occur in terms of access to social facilities by the government or public institutions, or by private institutions in education, housing and health, including common property resources like water bodies, grazing land and other lands of common use. Sometimes when the pattern of stigma and discrimination is broken, it is possible for someone to suffer stigma but not discrimination, for example, when legislation prevents stigmatized groups, such as an ethnic minority, being treated differently from other members of society. Any attempt to reduce stigma may reinforce it, for example, when university quotas are reserved for members of underprivileged communities, others resent and find ways of discriminating.

Attempts to analyse stigma and discrimination have led to narrower definitions that are not always universally understood, such as the distinction between 'felt' and 'enacted' stigma (Jacoby, 1994; Scrambler & Hopkins, 1986; UNAIDS, 2001). Felt stigma—which has also been referred to as self-stigmatization and as fear of stigma—refers to the expectations of stigmatized individuals as to how others will react to their condition. Felt stigma leads people to hide their stigmatizing condition, if it is possible, which limits the extent to which they experience discrimination. Meanwhile, enacted stigma is defined as the actual experience of stigma and discrimination.

In the last two decades, many developing countries have enacted laws to prevent discriminatory practices and to equalize opportunities for the physically challenged in employment, health and education. The People with Disabilities Act (1995) in India, the Disability Discrimination Act (2002) in Korea and the Human Rights and Equal Opportunity Commission Act (1986) in Australia are some of the examples of comprehensive legislative measures. Almost all developing countries now have disability-related laws to provide equal opportunity to people with disabilities in education, employment and other spheres. In a collectivist society, it is not only the disabled who get stigmatized but also their family and the support givers, making them vulnerable as well and reducing their capacity to provide support—emotional and of other kinds.

Poverty and Social Exclusion

Exclusion from society is a defining characteristic of both disability and poverty, and its causal consequences stem from a variety of factors, such as preoccupation with survival needs, lack of awareness and access to government schemes and denial of available services and infrastructure, including health, education, employment opportunities, legal system and so on. This exclusion is more pronounced in the case of people with disabilities, inasmuch as they are excluded from mainstream social, economic and political opportunities. As a consequence, people with disabilities and their families are frequently rendered into the ranks of the chronic poor (Eyben & Ferguson, 2000; Hulme, Moore & Shepherd, 2001). The UNESCO studies estimate that 98 per cent of children with disabilities in developing countries are denied formal education (Hegarty, 1995). As Elwan (1999) has noted that among these children, those who acquire education often receive inferior treatment, have low expectations of themselves, experience low expectations from their significant others and fail to get the support they need to participate equally. As adults, discrimination also tends to exclude them from employment and income-earning opportunities, leaving them in perpetual poverty (Hoogeveen, 2005; Lwanga-Ntale, 2003; Tudawe, 2001; World Bank, 2005). This initial exclusion and lack of growth opportunities create a downward cycle of economic well-being that can follow disabled people throughout their lives.

People with disabilities are historically excluded from the mainstream social life. In the traditional Indian society, they were integrated within the joint families and contributed towards collective family income by engaging in whatever economic activities they could. However, this family and community integration of the disabled which occurred was at maintenance level, where only the basic care was available to the people with disabilities (Dalal, 2000b). The disintegration of the traditional system and breaking down of joint families in India has created a serious problem of the social and economic rehabilitation of the population with disabilities. Urbanization and movement of population from rural to urban centres for jobs have affected the disabled people from the poor strata the most. Another factor which has significantly added to the existing exclusion is caste divide in India. The people from the lower castes form the major chunk of people below the poverty line in India. According to the 2001 Census of India, scheduled castes and tribes comprise 16.2 per cent and 8.2 per cent, respectively, of India's population. Roughly, 47.3 per cent of India's rural poor are concentrated in these groups. The proportions of rural SC and ST households below the poverty line were 30.1 per cent and 39.4 per cent respectively, as compared to a poverty rate of 17.7 per cent for rural non-scheduled households. Radhakrishnan, Rao, Ravi and Reddy (2006) estimated the index of chronic poverty from the data of 55th round of NSS (National Sample Survey of India) and found that 34.1 per cent of the SCs and 32.8 per cent of the OBCs were chronically poor. These data show that

India's most socially excluded castes are the poorest of the poor. There are no national data but one can conjecture that the largest chunk of India's disabled fall in these two caste categories.

The social exclusion of lower castes from the mainstream community life is based on the concept of purity and pollution where these castes were till recent past treated as untouchables. This exclusion is still embedded in the societal relations and societal institutions—the process through which individuals or groups are wholly or partially excluded from full participation in the society in which they live (Haan, 1997), resulting in deprivation and poverty. Sen (2000) has differentiated between 'active and passive exclusion'. He defines active exclusion as exclusion through the deliberate policy interventions by the government, or by other agencies, whereas passive exclusion is exclusion through the social processes in which there are no deliberate attempts to exclude them, but in effect these groups of people find themselves becoming victims of various forms of social exclusion.

The most telling effect of this exclusion is on educational opportunities that the disabled poor people have. As one can guess, the Indian scenario is dismal. The National Sample Survey Organisation (2004) found that 55 per cent of the disabled in India are illiterate; only 9 per cent have completed higher secondary education. Only 11 per cent of disabled people in the age group 5–18 years are enrolled in special schools in urban areas and in rural areas, it is less than 1 per cent. In August 2004, the NCPED put out a report titled *Research Study on Present Education Scenario*. According to its latest report (2015), only 0.56 per cent of disabled students were in higher education against 3 per cent reservation. These data are consistent with the overall scenario in the developing countries where about 90 per cent of children with disabilities do not go to school (EFA Global Monitoring Report, 2008).

This dismal scenario has to be seen in the light of the fact that the Government of India had started the scheme of integrated education for the disabled way back in 1974. It was a major shift in the government policy from special schools to integrated schools for providing education to the disabled children. Except for the severely handicapped, other handicapped children were to be integrated into the ordinary schools with the help of special teachers, aids and resources. Funds were made available to suitably modify the buildings to make them more accessible. In the International Decade of the Disabled (1993–2002), large funding was made available by the government and other agencies for this scheme. In later years, instead of effectively implementing scheme of integrated schools and engaging in the exercise of removing its lacuna, this scheme was disbanded, to be replaced by a new international catchword 'inclusion education', promoted by UN Convention on the Rights of the Child (1989), World Conference on Education for All (1990). Based on tempting ideals of 'right to education as a basic human right', 'learner-focused education' and 'improving the quality of education for all' inclusive education became the guiding principle for the formulation of educational policies in many developing countries (Centre for Studies in Inclusive Education [CSIE], 2004). How this policy change has brought qualitative change in the education of the poorest strata of the society is a contentious issue.

In the mid-1980s, community-based rehabilitation (CBR) was promoted as an alternative to the medical model of rehabilitation of people with disabilities with emphasis on inclusive social development. The emphasis in CBR is on social integration of its members with disability through locally generated support and resources. The local communities were encouraged to forge a common front to cope with the disadvantages of physical disability. This movement got impetus by a seminal publication by David Werner (2009, 2nd edition) *Disabled Village Children* which became a very popular compendium for community workers in providing rehabilitation services in remote areas. The compendium provides detailed information along with easy-to-implement strategies for the rehabilitation of children with disabilities by using locally available response.

CBR, in recent years, has become a major vehicle to augment physical, educational and vocational rehabilitation of the millions in developing countries (Sharma, 2007). Understanding cultural aspects of the community is the key to the success of any CBR programme. The factors, such as attitudes, beliefs and values prevalent in a community determine to a large extent the status of disabled people in that community, the integration of people with disability in the social mainstream and the way in which the community takes up the responsibility of their rehabilitation. A systematic understanding of these cultural factors was essential to plan CBR activities. In the 1980s and 1990s, CBR was promoted throughout the Asian and African countries as the most viable programme, though in later years, it lost its momentum and popular support. CBR as a movement did not succeed in India and continued only in a small pocket with government and international aid. Evaluation study of seven large CBR programmes in different parts of the country did not provide an encouraging picture (Dalal, 2000b). These CBR programmes flawed due to the glossy-unrealistic Western view of local communities as cohesive working units and due to the centralized planning of rehabilitation activities. In a joint policy paper, ILO, UNESCO and WHO (2004) have brought out a new version of CBR. This new version attempts to manoeuvre CBR towards the current jargon of poverty alleviation, and to align it with the Millennium Development Goals. We learnt no lessons from the failure of community development programmes of the 1950s and 1960s (Jain, Krishnamurthi & Tripathi, 1985) and failure of Panchayati Raj scheme (Department of Rural Development, 1985).

The evidence converging from many surveys and analyses of existing policies and structures suggest that exclusion is the main link between impairment and disability and between disability and poverty. Exclusion from public infrastructure tends to limit the availability of sanitation, clean water, electricity and health care services. These limitations tend to increase the risk of further impairment, creating a mutually reinforcing cycle (Yeo & Moore, 2003). The findings do not merely indicate the power of exclusion to create both poverty and disability. The review presented here also illustrates how government policies leading to inclusion and empowerment can result in turnaround and can severe the causal links between poverty and disability and thus, set the conditions for their upward mobility. The critical factor is the augmentation of visibility and participation of people with disabilities in social and economic spheres.

It is important to note that impairment does not lead directly to disability. Impairment becomes a disability in a specific social context (often because society does not respect the needs and the rights of citizens living with impairment). Exclusion mutes the collective ability of disabled populations to express their needs, and thus allows society to design physical and social environments where impairments become disabilities. In the long run, it leads to the establishment of institutions, attitudes and environments that advertently or inadvertently restrict the choices of people with impairments.

The extent of a person's disability, therefore, may not necessarily be a natural consequence of his or her impairment, but may, instead, be exacerbated by exclusion or by a sole consequence of exclusion. This finding is supported by work of the ILO (2002), which asserts, among other things, that "the lack of mobility or the inability to speak or to see was not a disability, the lack of education and vocational training certainly is." Since exclusion is the primary link between impairment and disability, further analysis of the model could suggest that exclusion is also the primary mechanism connecting causal elements of impairment and poverty.

Lack of Access: Disability-unfriendly Physical Environment

One of the reasons that exacerbate exclusion of the disabled people from the civic life is the poor accessibility of public places. Though central and state governments in India have repeatedly pledged that public buildings would be made accessible for the disabled people, the situation has only marginally improved. Ramps or lifts that accommodate wheelchairs, signs in Braille, audio commands at traffic signals or toilets that wheelchair-bound people can use are still rare sights, and in rural areas, they are almost non-existent. Buses and trains are virtually out of bounds for people in wheelchairs. Various physical access audit reports have come to the same conclusion. This lack of accessibility also has serious implications for the education of children with disabilities. Most of the regular schools are out of their reach. There is hardly any transport facility, proper approach roads or toilets in schools which children with disabilities can use. Even special schools in the rural areas are for namesake, hardly imparting any worthwhile education. Despite all big talks about inclusive education, funds which are spent for creating disability-friendly schools in the *Sarva Shiksha Abhiyan* (Universal Education Scheme) are less than 1 per cent of the total annual budget of primary education of the Central Government in 2008. Right to Education Act (2009) has many provisions for the inclusive education of children with disabilities. However, no effective mechanism is stipulated to assess the special needs of such children. Only, the time will show however effective provisions of this Act will be in the schooling of children with disabilities.

The same is the story of vocational training programmes. The poor with disabilities are thus not unemployed but are rendered unemployable. The situation of women with disability is even worse. There is a critical need to build an enabling psychological and physical environment that is supportive of the ability of the woman with a disability to function, within the limits caused by the disability itself, as an equal member of the society.

This is the scenario in spite of some landmark legislative developments, such as the Persons with Disability Act (1995) and the National Trust Act (2002). In spite of the laws that were enacted and the schemes that the government has initiated, the situation is far worse in case of MNCs with only 0.05 per cent of their workforce constituting disabled people. One can guess that employment of rural people with disabilities would be almost negligible.

It can be further noted that, in India, the gap between the employment of the disabled and that of non-disabled people is widening. The majority of persons with disability in India are capable of productive work. Despite the fact, the employment rate of the disabled population is lower (about 60 per cent on average) than the general population, with the gap widening since the 1990s. Having a disability reduces the probability of being employed by over 30 per cent for males in rural Uttar Pradesh and Tamil Nadu though the effect is lower for women. Around 45 per cent of households which have a person with a disability report that an adult in the family misses, on average, 2.5 hours of every day work to take care of the [disabled] member. However, other adult men in the same household are more likely to be working due to the need to compensate for lost income (World Bank Report, 2008).

Despite the most optimistic outlook for change in employment opportunities for women with disabilities, the present reality is that the best hope for productive work may lie in self-employment, probably on a cooperative basis with others. Apart from economic independence, work is an essential means of enabling a person to develop a sense of identity and self-esteem. Thus, gainful employment is an important means of promoting the social integration of disabled women.

Rural Employment

Employment of the rural poor has ostensibly taken the centre stage in the contemporary thinking on disability in India emphasized by planners, policy-makers and disability organizations. With the rural economy in decline, nearly 40 per cent of the household have no land of their own and it is estimated that the rural unemployment is as high as 30 per cent. The government schemes of the Rural Employment and Rajiv Gandhi Rojagar Yojna, which are now amalgamated into the National Rural Employment Guarantee Scheme (NREGS), are supposed to focus on the unemployed with disabilities as a special group. Under this scheme, one member of each poor household is guaranteed 100 days' work. The work is mostly unskilled hard labour with wages up to ₹100 per day. Obviously, only a few partially disabled persons can opt for such work. The number of disabled beneficiaries in the NREGS was only 167,934 (about 0.1 per cent) against 16 million beneficiaries as on January 2007. Inclusive development and employment is still a distant dream for poor people with disabilities despite grand schemes and tall promises which the consecutive governments keep making.

Major Legal and Policy Initiatives

In the last two decades, the Government of India took some major steps to deal with the massive challenge of physical and mental disability. Apart from various schemes, concessions and programmes, the government has taken major legal measures to mainstream the people with disabilities. Some of these legal and policy initiatives which have implications for improving health and well-being of poor with disabilities are as listed here.

The Rehabilitation Council of India Act, 1992

This Act was enacted in line with the Medical Council of India Act in the field of disability. It led to the establishment of the Rehabilitation Council of India (RCI). The RCI is responsible for standardizing and monitoring training courses for rehabilitation professionals, granting recognition to institutions running courses and maintaining a Central Rehabilitation Register of rehabilitation professionals. The RCI Act was amended in 2000 to give the RCI an additional responsibility of promoting research in the fields of rehabilitation and special education.

The Persons with Disabilities (Equal Opportunities, Protection of Rights and Full Participation) Act, 1995

This Act, for the first time, provided a legal framework for persons with disabilities and protected their rights. It lays down what education and employment opportunities must be created for the disabled, stipulates the creation of barrier-free access to public places and public transport and supports the right of disabled persons to live independent lives.

The National Trust Act, 1999

This Act provides for the constitution of a national body for the welfare of people with autism, cerebral palsy, mental retardation and multiple disabilities. The Act mandates the promotion of measures for the care and protection of persons with these disabilities in the event of the death of their parents, procedures for appointment of guardians and trustees for persons in need of such protection and support to registered organizations to provide need-based services in times of crisis to the families of the disabled.

The National Policies for Persons with Disabilities, 2005

This Act recognizes that persons with disabilities are the valuable human resource for the country and seeks to create an environment that provides equal opportunities to them, protection of their rights and full participation in society. The focus of the policy is on the prevention, early detection and rehabilitation and education and employment of the persons with disabilities.

The Right to Education (RTE) Act, 2009

The Act is commonly known as RTE Act and was finally passed by the parliament on 26 August 2009 (notified on 16 February 2010 to come into effect from 1 April 2010). This act puts the responsibility of ensuring enrolment, attendance and completion on the government. The RTE Act tries to safeguard the rights of the children belonging to the disadvantaged groups and the weaker sections, protect them from any kind of discrimination and ensure their completion of elementary education. Children with disabilities have been included in the definition of the child belonging to a disadvantaged group. The Act mandates for private unaided and specified category of schools to admit at least 25 per cent of its entry level class from children belonging to weaker and disadvantaged groups.

This Act has, in fact, remodelled the concept of the integrated school in its overarching philosophy of inclusive education in which the emphasis is on bringing change in the school environment for effective integration of disabled children. Accordingly, the new policy of the government focuses on improving physical access, developing infrastructure and focusing on special needs and awareness programme.

The Rights of Persons with Disability Bill, 2014

This proposed Bill aims to replace the Persons with Disabilities (Equal Opportunities, Protection of Rights and Full Participation) Act, 1995. Instead of seven disabilities specified in the Act, the Bill covers 19 conditions. Persons with at least 40 per cent of a 'disability' are entitled to certain benefits such as reservations in education and employment, preference in government schemes and so on. The Bill confers several rights and entitlements to disabled persons. These include disabled friendly access to all public buildings, hospitals, modes of transport, polling stations and so on. This Bill is yet be passed by the Parliament.

A perusal of the disability-related legal provisions (and the new bill) suggests that they have many common features. One, they all have been framed keeping in view the medical model, that is, defining disability in terms of orthopaedic, neural and physical impairment. Social and community-based models of disability are not taken into consideration. Two, these acts are modelled on the UN Charter and disability organization having their base in the Western world, unmindful of the Indian conditions and constraints. Rooted in individual-focused perspective of rehabilitation, these laws ignore interdependence and connectedness of social life in India. The rhetoric of right-based approach borrowed from the West has become a by-word for disability-lobbyists and law-makers. These legislations take no cognizance of Indian reality, social beliefs and practices and poverty. Three, disability acts are very ambitious; while trying to achieve a wide range of goals, they sometimes try to achieve a higher level of goals but fail to meet some of the basic goals. In a country where basic access is denied to more than 90 per cent of the population with the disability, mostly poor living in slums or small towns, talking of equal opportunities and quality of life is utopian. The laws show dreams which have no connection with the realities of life and are unachievable. Four, the most problematic in these acts is the casual approach to monitoring and evaluation. The acts and schemes look impressive on paper but remains on paper in most of the cases. They rarely achieve the goals and only promote tokenism and nothing changes in reality. Without effective implementation and accountability on the part of government agencies, these laws only remain good showpieces. The implementation of these legal provisions is often left to the state governments who lack in resources, manpower and monitoring system.

Rise and Fall of Disability Movement

Till today, NGOs in the field of rehabilitation are registered under the Indian Society Act, 1860 and the Public Charitable Trust Act of the Central Government which is modified from time to time, the latest version enacted in 2013. Whatever public service these NGOs offer for people with disabilities, these are still covered under the umbrella term 'charity'. As such, many rehabilitation policies, programmes and practices of the British India were perpetuated by the Indian government. The situation started changing when the concept of charity was replaced with that of 'welfare' after India's independence. The country under the influence of Nehruvian socialism took upon itself the onerous responsibility of providing rehabilitation services to one and all. It led to the growth of centralized and institutionalized services for the welfare of the people with disabilities in the first decade of Independence. Many laws were enacted and welfare programmes and schemes were launched. The government established national and state-level institutions in different corners of the country, specializing in physical and mental disabilities. These institutions were supposed to serve as the nodal agencies to feed to local bodies throughout the country (Dalal, 2011). The paternalistic attitudes in its new form continued to influence the functioning of the government organizations and other welfare agencies. Such an attitude was very much evident in camp-culture and free-distribution of aids and appliances by the government agencies. Given the massive problem of disability in the country, these sporadic efforts hardly made any dent.

The three developments of the 1980s brought significant change in this scenario. First, the Government of India became a signatory of the WHO declaration of 'Health for All by the Year 2000' and committed to 'Rehabilitation to All'. Many international and regional agencies put in enormous resources and in a short time, rehabilitation of the people with disability became a major national programme. Second, under the new policy, the government entrusted the NGOs to shoulder the much greater responsibility of providing rehabilitation services. The whole idea was that these NGOs will be more committed and accountable to the cause they are working for. The third change was greater emphasis on community-based rehabilitation as a strategy to reach all those who need these services. It was realized that institutional services were reaching to only 2–3 per cent of the needy population and there was no possibility of radically expanding the coverage of these services. The other viable option was to encourage local communities to shoulder a greater responsibility of planning and implementing the programmes and to generate additional resources. CBR philosophy and practices are already discussed in the preceding section. In the 1900s, the Government of India adopted CBR as its official programmes to be implemented throughout the country. In the beginning of the millennia, the disability movement throughout the world as well as in India weakened and with that, CBR also declined. Williams (2003) has conjectured that in the West, the governments dole out a series of disability benefits, which as a result, weakened disability movement. Lack of support from the Western NGOs and governments had its effect on disability funding and enthusiasm in the developing world as well (Vyas, 1998).

Culture and Community Participatory

In the disability sector, schemes, plans and practices are guided by the ideology, interest and experience of European and North American agencies which are incidentally the major source of funding of poverty and disability projects in India and other developing countries. During the final quarter of the twentieth century, Westerners have poured in (or trickled in) their well-intentioned aid, riding on the support and enthusiasm of Asian professionals. In the 1970s, Western aid agencies were funding special schools and were engaged in the training of developmental professionals, project staff and specialized teachers in India. In the 1980s, with the government opening up its doors to international agencies, much of the developmental planning of governments and local NGOs was influenced by ideology and vision of the rich countries. Unmindful of the local traditions, practices and beliefs, programmes fabricated in the West were implemented in the developing world. Most of these programmes centred on community participation as the major goal. Brand new schemes with catchy rhetoric, such as normalization, integration, community-based rehabilitation and equal participation were transported and offered with funding. In the 1990s, the buzz words were inclusion, social model, partnership and disability rights (Miles, 2000).

Proponents of these new initiatives most often avoid mentioning that the new concept is a very recent experiment with no working models, no independent evaluations and no basis in Asian cultures and history. Nobody bothers to explain that concepts, like CBR, are premised on an urban idealization of rural 'community spirit', where everyone is supposed to fulfil their duty of caring for one another. Simultaneously, urban disabled peoples' groups are being taught to fight for 'disability rights' based on a Euro-American male concept of the autonomous individual owing no duty to anyone but himself. These packages are being framed as universal solutions (Miles, 2000) for the rehabilitation of people with disability in poor countries. It may be mentioned here that community models of rehabilitation are rarely promoted by the developed countries as solutions in their own set-up.

A further question arises concerning the appropriateness and applicability of the Western-based notion of empowerment, which presupposes that rights are exercised and that decisions are made in accordance with the preferences and wishes of the individual in developing countries. Such an individualized notion of empowerment, as espoused by the international disability movement, runs contrary to accepted social customs and practices that are found in many developing countries. In societies such as India, it is customary that all major decisions, for example, who one should marry, the purchase of property and career choice, are taken not by the individual, but generally made collectively through consultation with the extended family and kinship networks (Lang, 1998). Participation thus has a different connotation in traditional societies.

The fact remains that unless active participation of the poor with disabilities is ensured, no significant change is expected in the present disability–poverty nexus. Dreze and Sen (2002) have argued for an instrumental and intrinsic significance of participation. Their plea is that democratic participation is essential in the Indian context where feudal mindsets still prevail. Dalal, Kumar and Gokhale (2000) found in their evaluation study of CBR programmes that community participation was generally low when the programme was seen as imposed from outside. In an extensive evaluation study of 15 social sector schemes in two districts (Saharanpur and Varanasi) of Uttar Pradesh, Pant and Pandey (2004) noted that the main cause of the poor implementation of the schemes was low involvement of programme functionaries, particularly of the beneficiaries. It is ironical that most of the governmental and non-governmental programmes emphasize on the active participation of the targeted population, in practice, they rarely have any say in planning, implementation and evaluation of such programmes. Most of these programmes are, in essence, repackaging of charity and welfare schemes of the earlier times. These programmes cultivate and sustain a culture of dependence by engaging in rituals and rhetoric of participation that masks the real intentions of the vested interest. Most of the disability NGOs are dependent on the government grants for sustenance and, therefore, rarely contest this state of affairs.

A New Model of Participatory Rehabilitation

This chapter views rehabilitation from a developmental perspective. Active participation of people with disabilities in a socio-economic programme is considered as an essential precondition for their social mainstreaming. A schematic model of disability–poverty nexus and participation–development as way-out is presented in Figure 5.1. As the model shows, disability and poverty have the propensity to get into a vicious cycle, mutually reinforcing each other, rendering the poor with disabilities as the most disadvantaged group in the society. Their participation in the developmental programmes is suppressed by

Figure 5.1:
Disability–poverty trap and upward mobility through active participation

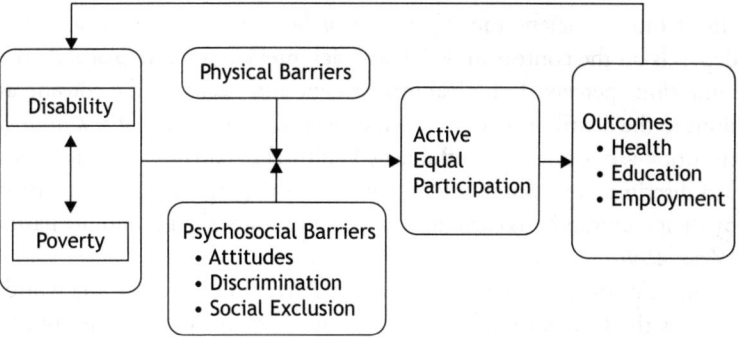

Source: Dalal (2010).

social exclusion and physical barriers. Consequently, they are low on all three indices of socio-economic development—health, education and employment. The model posits that breaking psychosocial and physical barriers is essential to facilitate the active and equal participation of the poor with disability in social and economic activities, and consequent upward mobility.

Development through participation is held as the most practical strategy by national and international agencies working on disability projects. They profess the democratic ideal of development—by the people, for the people and of the people. As a tool of development, participation aims to transform, connect and give a sense of belonging to people. Many experiments are going on in the field to augment the participation of the poorest strata of the society in developmental programmes. Despite so much of emphasis and awareness, participation of the poor (and disabled) is an unrealized goal in most of the developmental projects. It is a major challenge for social scientists and activists to build the knowledge base, expertise and experience to figure out why participation has failed despite all noises made about it. We need to know what will work. This chapter has shed light on psychosocial and physical barriers which complicate active participation of the poor with disabilities. Many of these barriers have built up on and been sustained by centuries old social, religious and economic edifice which still serve the purpose of many vested-interest groups in the society. The poorest among the poor are struggling against all odds to lead a life with dignity.

Culture shapes the meaning and implications of psychosocial barriers and participation of the people with disability. For example, in hierarchical Indian society, the experience of belonging and discrimination depends on the context in which a social interaction takes place. At the same time, perceived physical impairment and need may be considerations in the distribution of economic reward. If the norms of reward distribution are according to established cultural practices, people may not feel discriminated. Sometimes a sense of belonging and being accepted by their community is considered more important than economic parity (Vyas, 1998).

Some of the new socio-economic initiatives in the developing world, such as the formation of self-help groups (SHGs) and capacity-building programmes, have actually renewed hopes of breaking the vitiating nexus between poverty and disability. Though most of the SHGs primarily engage in micro-financing—in saving and credit activities, the very fact of working together promotes the spirit of participation. About 80 per cent of the SHGs comprise poor women though the poorest ones are mostly left out. According to the National Policy for Persons with Disability announced in February 2006, the government intends to promote projects where the representation of women with disability is at least 25 per cent of the total beneficiaries. The government encourages the disabled people to form SHGs to engage in efforts to provide community-based support services through mutual support mechanisms and advocacy for disabled persons to achieve their maximum potential and assume responsibility for their own lives.

Joining SHGs has resulted in the empowerment of these women, who, through their improved economic status and experience of collective self-management of SHGs, have acquired visibility and voice in the household as well as in the community. Other positive outcomes experienced by SHG members relate to increase in self-worth, communication skills, better dealing with problem situations and a decrease in family violence (Tankha, 2002). Similarly, the large-scale capacity-building programmes have intended to prepare people to manage developmental projects as partners and stakeholders. ADD–India (Action for Disability and Development–India, located in Bangalore) is one of the major organizations which is promoting SHGs in South India through capacity-building training. In a unique scheme of SHGs started by the government of Tamil Nadu, rural poor below the poverty line are encouraged to form groups in which at least 20 per cent members are disabled and need all kinds of special assistance. The evaluation report suggests that more than 21,000 such groups were formed in 2005–2006 in different districts (Directorate of Town Panchayats, 2008, Activities of Empowerment). Taken together, these two initiatives have succeeded in giving rise to a new awakening in the poorest strata of the society. Poor people are learning to collectively raise their voice about their rights and stake in the growing economy.

One important way to augment active participation is to make developmental programmes compatible with local beliefs, practices and aspirations. India has a long tradition of community participation in social and religious activities, which needs to be harnessed for the developmental work. Socio-spiritual beliefs of the community which bind members together can be harnessed for socio-economic development also. Although some care and caution need to be exercised in dealing with religious institutions whose primary motto is charity and welfare, not participation. The point is that once a programme strikes a positive cord with people's feelings and faith, it gathers its own momentum. Such programmes are self-evolving and self-sustaining. Participation is a problem when a programme with a rigid structure is imposed from outside. The phenomenal success of the *Swadhyaya* movement in western India is a good example of how a programme can thrive on local beliefs and social practices. The Swadhyaya is a socio-spiritual movement for self-development and social transformation (Giri, 1998) in which community work is considered as *bhakti* (worship), where skills and labour are taken as offerings to the Lord. The Swadhyaya aims to uphold equality and dignity of all human beings, sharing of resources, concern for general well-being and endeavours for the growth and development of the community (Shah, Seth & Visaria, 1998). Presently, the Swadhyaya movement has a following of more than 3 million people, spread over 20,000 villages. It has a disciplined cadre known as *Swadhyayees* involved in a variety of programmes and activities, geared for individual and social development. The Swadhyaya has the ideology of active participation of all community members, including people with disabilities in planning its activities. It offers a unique model of socio-economic development through community participation in spiritual activities. Though it is a socio-spiritual movement of poor communities, it can be easily adapted in the case of disability rehabilitation.

The contention is that there is no one best way to ensure participation of poor with disabilities in developmental activities, nor can it be achieved through a single intervention. Participation builds on trust in implementing agencies over a period of time and sustains on positive results. Psychosocial barriers cannot be wished away and knowing that attitudes and beliefs have the tenacity to persist, participation is a slow process to achieve health, education and education-related goals of development. There are no shortcuts, nor any band-aid type of approach work. In fact, such shortcut approaches yield quick results in the short run but do more damage than good in the long run. People feel cheated. Participation cannot be ensured or imposed from outside by the funding and implementing agencies; it is a natural, spontaneous and evolving process when a programme is owned by the people for whom it is intended. It is in this context that participatory development possesses a major challenge for social scientists and activists as well as for poor with disabilities.

In this context, it is pertinent to ask whose ideal we are striving to achieve through these developmental programmes. As noted by Tripathi and Sinha (2013), all psychosocial-economic interventions have a vision of the society and they programme their activities to realize that vision. These visions or ideals are often based on the implicit beliefs about human conditions and the goals they cherish to accomplish. It is, therefore, important to understand implicit theories which interventionists carry in their mind and which get manifested in participatory development programmes. A sustained participation can be ensured only if it is based on a common vision of all stakeholders and which is compatible with changing times (Dalal, 2010). Participation of people with disability and their families has to be viewed as agents of change, not merely as recipients. Right-based approaches many times lead to confrontation and competition ripping the very social cohesiveness which ensures integration and empowerment of all sections of the local communities. There has to be space and opportunities for experimenting with different participatory models as just one model cannot be best for all.

6

Methodological Imperatives for Cultural Psychology of Health

For the rapidly expanding field of cultural psychology of health, methodological challenges are enormous. The field has expanded to include the physical, social, psychological and spiritual well-being of people, and also human strengths, resilience and happiness. In the Indian as well as other traditional societies, health and healing are considered integral to the general well-being. Healing aims to restore harmony and balance within the individual through a symbiosis of the body, the mind and the spirit. All socio-cultural aspects of human life, in some way, figure within the holistic conceptualization of wellness and well-being.

The research methodologies which are employed in psychology and other social sciences are pertinent as long as the illness model of health is the subject matter of investigation. But as we expand the domain of research to include suffering, healing, pain, freedom, happiness and so on, we face a methodological challenge of bigger magnitude. It calls for expanding the repertoire of research methods to address new questions or the old ones framed differently. These new domains of research call for research methodologies which are more holistic in nature, not in terms of fragmented variables and their measures. Second, most of the research methods employed in psychological research are appropriate for doing research on the 'other' person, where a dichotomy between researcher and respondent is clearly maintained. In this paradigm, the respondent is merely a data provider, and the data is processed by the researcher to draw conclusions about the 'other' person(s). Participatory and self-administered research obviously needs a different kind of methodological approach, and many such methodologies are still evolving in psychology. The research in which participants are actively involved in intervention, interpretation and appraisal of the outcomes, as in the case of chronic diseases, needs a different type of research methodology. Third, the scientific psychology of health can significantly benefit from Indian methodologies of yoga and meditation, developed and used to understand the human body, mind and consciousness. These self-administered methodologies can be of help, not only in dealing with physical and mental health challenges but also in self-transformation of people to a higher level of functioning.

Health psychology emanated as a separate field of research from social psychology in the 1980s and focused on psychosocial aspects of health and illness (Taylor, 2006). As a sub-branch of social psychology, it employed the positivistic methods of its parent discipline. Cultural psychology of health as an independent field has a short history of past 2–3 decades. For this newly emerging discipline, it is a research in a daunting proposition when health practices and beliefs prevalent in different cultures are brought within the subject field of health psychology. Folk and faith healings are also brought within the subject field of health research, as are the practices of yoga and meditation. This complicates the research scenario and poses a major challenge of finding appropriate methods which can juxtapose different healing traditions. Cultural psychology of health is open to borrowing methods from different cultures and disciplines. Research methods used in cultural anthropology and sociology are widely employed to make across and within culture comparisons. Indigenous psychologies can also potentially contribute to identifying and developing new research methodologies to understand the phenomena which are considered mystical and esoteric by the mainstream psychology (Watts, 1975). Smith has discussed the decolonizing of research methodologies to understand health practices of indigenous societies (Smith, 2012). The challenge of finding appropriate methodologies for cultural psychology of health is leading to many innovations and breakthroughs.

It is to be mentioned here that rather than discussing methods of research, in this chapter, we are focusing on research (or scientific) methodologies. In brief, the methodology is defined as the *science of methods*—ontology, epistemology and rationale of a method employed in a research project. In other words, the methodology is about the rationale and principles that guide our research practices. Methodology explains and justifies the use of certain methods or tools in our specific research project. It entails philosophical assumptions that underlie any natural, social or human science project. Often such assumptions are implicit in the kind of methods we are using and rarely articulated. Simply put, methodology refers to what counts as the knowledge (McGregor & Murnane, 2010); methods are the tools, techniques and procedures followed to conduct research. Surveys, interviews, participant observation, experiments and so on are examples of methods, not of methodology which is an umbrella term for a class of methods. In this chapter, methods, per se, are not discussed, which can be found in most of the textbook on health psychology. Our focus in this chapter is on methodologies as they are integral part of research paradigm, or in a broader sense, part of a knowledge tradition which may vary from culture to culture. Kuhn (1970) placed positive science as a premium research paradigm which psychology borrowed from natural science. In social sciences other paradigms have evolved in recent history, subscribing to different research methodologies and methods. The chapter deliberates on different methodological schemes of classifying methods of research, and on their salience for making sense of health, healing and well-being.

Culture and knowledge traditions are closely interwoven as culture provides the context within which methods of knowing make sense. In the larger domain of health and well-being, the obtained results cannot be separated from the methodology of research. This is the reason that each of the Indian system of healing—Ayurveda, yoga and meditation and indigenous practices—has developed its own methodology to implicate the research findings. The chapter highlights Indian methods of knowing and points at the need to innovate in the area of research methodology.

Methodologies of Modern Psychology

Wilhelm Wundt, the German psychologist, is remembered for establishing the first psychology laboratory at Leipzig in 1889. Psychology students are made to remember this historical place and the date by heart and are taught how experiments were conducted in his laboratory to study the structure of human consciousness. Wundt used the introspection method to take the verbal report of the experimental subject to know about their conscious reaction to stimulus conditions. In this, subjects were presented with well-defined and tightly controlled stimuli and instructed to provide—deliberate and immediate observation of inner processes (Wundt, 1888; cited in Hatfield, 2005)—the experiences that are prompted by stimuli. It was aimed to compare different subjects' introspective reports as prompted by the same stimuli. Prior to conducting the experiments, subjects were trained to give as truthful report as possible. In fact, subjects used to be senior members of the research team who had better articulation and skills to report their immediate experience. However, the introspection method was considered too subjective for an objective science of psychology and was completely abandoned when psychology moved to the United States. A new school of behaviourism took over, with a more rigorous experimental approach. This is also no surprise that the first department of psychology established in India at the Calcutta University was the Department of Experimental Psychology.

For almost a century, psychology was obsessed to establish its scientific credentials. To be a science, it borrowed the experimental methods of physical sciences from physics, chemistry and biology, established laboratories and attempted to conduct experiments under controlled conditions. The hallmarks of such experimental research were—objectivity, control, replicability and validity. Experimental psychologists aspired to have the same degree of rigour in conducting experiments on human beings, as physicists have on inanimate objects. The experimental method became the most popular method in almost all branches of psychology and remained so for next 60–70 years.

Research methodology in psychology expanded to include testing, measurement, observation, surveys, case studies and so on. Objectivity, control, replicability and validity remained the criteria for evaluating these methods. This emphasis on objectivity makes sense from a psychological science standpoint that emphasizes theoretically driven research and replicability of research procedures and design. Psychological knowledge multiplied rapidly using these diverse methods. In psychological research and teaching, basic knowledge of these methods is considered essential. These methods of research are presumed to distinguish psychology from humanities and philosophy, as well as from other social sciences, such as sociology and anthropology. Psychology is considered to be the most scientific of all social sciences.

From the very first introductory course, students are taught that psychology is a science because it relies on the methods of science to test hypotheses and to generate new knowledge. Teaching research methods is a major component of course curriculum in psychology at the undergraduate, postgraduate and higher levels. Research methods are emphasized both in theory and practical classes. No training in psychology is considered to be complete until a student acquires proficiency both in experimental and non-experimental methods and can use these methods for testing psychological theories and propositions. When health psychology started growing as a separate branch in the 1980s, these methods of the mainstream psychology became the obvious choice in research studies.

We need to understand Western psychologist's obsession to be a scientist in the historical context. Four centuries back, Europe was emerging from the Dark Age into the age of Enlightenment. It was the time when science was struggling to free itself from the powerful control of the church and was trying to establish itself on an empirical foundation. Descartes made a valiant effort to demarcate the domains of science and religion, those which were subjective, mystical, metaphysical and immeasurable were considered the legitimate fields of study for the church and religion. The ones which could be measured and were empirically verifiable came under the domain of science. He laid down the foundation of modern science which subsequently led to the emergence of modern psychology. This modern psychology, which was built on the work of Comte, Popper, Kuhn and others, left out the human psyche to be taken care of by religion and sensory-conscious experiences, and observable behaviour to be the legitimate field of scientific inquiry. The methodology of the science of psychology thus developed on the premise of a material—physical human existence and studying objective—measurable behaviour (Gower, 1997). The purpose of such a research was to understand, control and change human behaviour. This positivistic science of psychology expanded and covered all the domains of psychological research.

Emic and Etic Approaches

Cultural psychology makes a distinction between 'emic' and 'etic' approaches to health and well-being. These two approaches refer to whether the cultural phenomenon is studied from inside or from outside. When the insider perspective is taken, it is called emic approach, and when the outsider perspective is taken it is called etic approach (Berry, 1989). The emic approach would, for example, focus on how people within a culture understand the meaning of health and well-being, perceive the causes of their illness, seek treatment, strive to improve their health status and so on. The etic approach would be concerned about the universality of such cultural response to health, how similar behaviour is observed across different cultures. Etic approach strives to develop health measures which can be used by different cultures. Etic knowledge refers to generalizations about human behaviour that are considered universally true. Although emics and etics are oftentimes regarded as in conflict and in research, one has to prefer one over the exclusion of the other, though complementarities of these two approaches to cultural psychology research is also recognized. The emic perspective is more relevant to comprehend and appreciate the nuances of a particular culture unless one resides within that culture. An outsider's (etic) perspective can never fully capture what it really means to be part of the culture.

When a comparison is to be made across cultures, the etic approach is not feasible, often imposed etics are used for such comparisons. Imposed etics are presumed or derived etics, taking emics of a particular culture. In reality, these are the emics of the Western culture which, with some cultural modification, are taken to establish the cross-cultural universality of Western theories and concepts. Use of positivistic methodologies fosters such false sense of universality.

Cultural and indigenous psychologies have built on etic approaches. From cultural psychology of health perspective, the study of folk health practices is mostly based on emic approach. Adair (2006) described different stages of indigenous psychologies across the world. He considered that the greater the cultural difference from the American context and the less developed the discipline, such as in Asia, the greater would be the need for indigenization of the discipline. By indigenization, he meant adding cultural content in Western theories in which etic and emic approaches are integrated. This position is contentious and is seen as an attempt to the adaptation of Western theories in different cultures.

Changing Paradigms of Research

All research presupposes a world view which is at the care of its research design, data collection and interpretation of the findings. In the philosophy of science, the concept of the paradigm has commonly been used when referring to theoretical assumptions and structures of science. In practice, the paradigm in a single piece of research can be defined by asking the following five basic questions (Denzin & Lincoln, 2005):

1. **Ontological:** What constitute health and well-being, nature of human existence, conception of society and social reality?
2. **Epistemological:** What constitutes new knowledge? Ways of knowing about health?
3. **Methodological:** Assumptions, relevance and applicability of the method used.
4. **Ethical:** Procedure of data collection; human dignity and privacy; who will benefit from this research?
5. **Practical:** Feasibility, efficiency of research.

A scientific paradigm evolves as an outcome of ongoing communication among the members of the scientific community over generations about the nature of science, its purpose, methods and accomplishments. It is over a period of time that a consensus emerges about what to research, how to conduct research and what to make of research findings? There are implicit assumptions and broad framework within which the research activities are supposed to be carried out. The research paradigm is sustained by building an environment and institutions for research, by educational programmes for students and young scholars. Commonly accepted theoretical assumptions, empirical generalizations and applications of research, as well as the methodology, technology and scientific language constitute what Kuhn (1970) called a 'paradigm'. A paradigm has a strong resistance to change. If there are findings that contradict a theory, the research community first tries to explain these 'anomalies' within the paradigm. If more anomalies arise, usually different groups of researchers try to modify the paradigm. Kuhn talked about revolutionary science when a new paradigm emerges with a new world view and set of principles of conducting research. For example, nuclear and quantum physics led to a new paradigm in physics, rejecting the mechanistic model of Newtonian physics.

Basically, positivistic–empirical research paradigm that psychology borrowed from the natural sciences remained the main basis of conducting research in psychology. Building on the materialistic–individualistic–capitalistic conception of the society, this research paradigm has thrived in psychology for almost a century. The mainstay of this paradigm is the experimental method but as mentioned earlier, other non-experimental methods were also added in the long run.

In positivistic methodologies, the empirical data forms the basis of inferring reality. In this paradigm, a distinction is made between the observer and the object of observation. The reality/truth is believed to be stable, predictable and knowable and independent of the observer. The scientific research methodology is believed to serve the purpose of approximating the essential truth of the subject matter under study. Experimentation, observation and testing are considered important to know the truth. Psychological reality is constructed 'out there', independent of any human perspective as if it could be known objectively through empirical observation (e.g., psychological test) and logical thinking by an 'external objective expert' (Parnas, Sass, & Zahavi, 2013).

If we scan the standard textbooks of psychology, most of the research reported in the area of cultural psychology of health is based on the positivistic scientific methods of research. Courses on scientific methods of research which the students are taught are primarily experimental and non-experimental methods within the positivistic tradition. Psychology students are given rigorous training in the use of these methods. It is only in the recent years that research in health psychology is getting exposed to alternative methods and other research paradigms. Research, taking the perspective of patients and caregivers, based on qualitative methods has brought about this change.

Alternative Paradigms

Many thinkers and researchers in the last 2–3 decades expressed doubts about the ideal of objectivity in psychology research, including James (1890) and Dilthey (1996). In more recent times, various critics have challenged the assumptions and methods of scientific psychology, ranging from social psychologists concerned about the ecological validity of experiments (Gergen, 1982; Rosenthal, 1976). Cultural, cross-cultural and indigenous psychologists have argued that psychology had normalized the behaviour of white middle-class-male under the auspices of objective science. Psychological phenomena are subjective in nature as they do not exist in the physical world. These are abstract concepts and operationalized for the purpose of conducting research. The meaning of these concepts may vary depending on the way they are understood in different cultures and theoretical framework. Objectification of such subjective phenomena by the researcher may be reflective of their cultural blinders (Goldberg, 1994). A good number of cultural phenomena cannot be translated from one culture to another. Objectivity remains a problematic notion in psychological research. Given that there is so much variation in the conceptualization of health and well-being, it is problematic to develop their measures which are universal in nature.

Though positivistic methodology still remains at the core of mainstream psychological science, many schools of thought and associated methodologies are posing a serious challenge to it. Some of the research paradigms which characterize academic psychology in the present times are listed here in a chronological order of their emergence. Here, only two prominent research paradigms are discussed. Some later paradigms, such as critical theory and deconstructionism, are part of the postmodernistic thinking about research and knowledge.

Phenomenological Paradigm

According to the phenomenological approach, people exist in the world as wakeful consciousness exists in the experiential world. Experience involves the dynamic engagement of the ego and focuses on positional consciousness and intentional relationship with the phenomenon. Phenomenology is, thus, a social theory of research which takes the position that the foundation of knowledge should be placed upon 'reality' as it could be consciously experienced (Smith, 2004).

Phenomenological paradigm began with Husserl (1859–1939), with emphasis on returning to the event or situation by attempting to gain understanding and interpretation from within. Husserl saw the individual as the focal point for social analysis and the originator of meaning. He argued that unless objects and events appeared to consciousness, it remains non-existent. To be cognized, it has to be cognized through someone's consciousness, where the consciousness is not just limited to awareness. In the broader sense, it will also include preconscious and unconscious processes. This paradigm of research was carried forward by Hegel and Heidegger in the twentieth century.

This paradigm takes the position that it is not possible to know the reality 'as such'. What we can know is the experiential reality, 'not' the experience of reality. Only experiential reality can be the valid subject matter of research. We can conduct studies to interpret human experiences.

Phenomenology aims to remain as faithful as possible to the phenomenon and to the context in which it appears in the world. It means that to study a particular phenomenon, a situation is sought in which individuals have first-hand experiences that they can describe as they actually took place in their life. The aim of a research is to capture the ways in which the phenomenon is experienced within the context.

Phenomenality certainly is a crucial fact for the domain of living beings. It would, for instance, surely be the case that an organism with a sonar system like the bat does not perceive what an organism equipped with a visual system like a man can perceive. The external world presumably looks very different to both. Similarly, though to a lesser extent, the experience of two individuals belonging to the same species can be expected to differ in their perception. Ricoeur (1970) terms theory-driven interpretations of personal experience, whether emanating from psychoanalytic, cognitive, discursive or other traditions.

In a way, all phenomenological data aim to be descriptive, often a distinction is made between descriptive phenomenology versus interpretive or hermeneutic, phenomenology. With descriptive (i.e., Husserl-inspired) phenomenology, it aims to reveal essential general meaning structures of a phenomenon. These researchers stay close to what is presented by the phenomenon in all its richness and complexity (Mohanty, 1988, cited in Giorgi, 1986, p. 9). Interpretive phenomenology, in contrast, has emerged from the work of hermeneutic philosophers, including Heidegger, Gadamer and Ricoeur, who argued that we have our embeddedness in the world of language and social relationships. Interpretation, thus, constitutes an inevitable and basic structure of our 'being-in-the-world'. Experience and interpretation thus cannot be separated. Taking a middle path, many prefer to see description and interpretation as a continuum where specific data may be of more or less interpretive nature (Finlay, 2009).

Social Constructionism

Social constructionism makes sense if we consider human beings not as a perceiver but as a conceiver of social and physical world. One must know before one can see. This approach holds that there is no truth or objectivity. The reality, as we see, is a mental and social construction. Our expectations, ideology and past knowledge determine what we see as real. Knowledge cannot be independent of the knower. Knowing the real world is an impossibility and always conjectural. The reality is constructed, structured and organized by the perceivers, which forms the basis for their subsequent behaviour. Berger and Luckmann (1966) have in their classic work *The Social Construction of Reality* stated that we see our everyday reality as ordered, structured and rational, and we take it for granted as natural. The language we use every day leads to the objectification of our presumptions against which we make sense of our percepts. We never realize that we are indeed living in a constructed world.

Social constructionism takes position that there are no truths or objective realities; all realities are socially constructed. We cannot directly describe our experiences, as all experiences are shaped by our construction of events. Scientific knowledge deals with these constructed realities—everyday subjective constructions on the part of people who are studied and scientific construction on the part of researcher in collecting, treating and interpreting data, as well as in the presentation of findings. If we extend this argument, all other forms of metatheory (including phenomenology, hermeneutics, realism and so on) are themselves constructions—socio-historically contingent and ideologically saturated. As Gergen (1985) stated that from a constructionist perspective, any attempt to test hypotheses about universal processes of the mind—cognition, motivation, perception, attitudes, prejudice, self-conception—seems to be misguided. These are social constructions, thus not subject to empirical evaluation outside a particular tradition of interpretation. The present research represents the arrogation of a uniquely Western ontology of the mind to the status of the universal.

The Quantitative and Qualitative Divide

In broad terms, all research methods can be classified into two categories—quantitative and qualitative methods—no matter which research paradigm is subscribed to. Research methodology before the modern age was qualitative in nature and remained so from the ancient time in all civilizations. Commentaries on classical and other texts often followed well laid out rules and practices in every society. Verbal reports used to be the basis of judging people and take important social–political–moral decisions. The interpretation used to be informal to deal with the practical matters and the modern concept of research as a formal–systematic–objective activity was not formulated. Students in Socrates' Academy and other schools, as well as in the ashrams of sages were taught to critique the verbal and written texts but its purpose was to understand its essence. Many of these methods are now considered mystical, esoteric, biased and, therefore, unscientific. In the initial phase, scientific psychology in Europe was close to what one would today call qualitative research. In this, verbal report of the 'experiences' by the subject used to be the main body of data. If one closely peruses the research done in Wundtian laboratories, one will notice that no clear distinction was made between qualitative and quantitative methods (e.g., Mays & Pope, 1995). Of course, the quantitative and qualitative methods that we employ in research today are, in a way, refinement of many centuries-old practices.

Scientific research has a preference for quantification ever since measurement was considered to be an essential requisite for scientific research. To establish its scientific credentials, psychological research emphasized quantification at all levels, taking quantification as akin to measurement. Positivistic psychology greatly emphasized development and use of tests, scales and measures in psychological research, including experimental research. Statistical techniques were extensively used to process these data, to test and develop psychological theories. Though psychoanalytic school popularized the case study method, there were few qualitative methods in psychology at that time. When in the 1980s and onwards, demand for qualitative methods increased in psychological research, and most of the methods were borrowed from other social sciences. In the last three decades, several new qualitative methods are developed in psychology. Two handbooks,

The Sage Handbook of Qualitative Research (2005, third edition) and *The Sage Handbook of Qualitative Research in Psychology* (2008), cover the whole range of qualitative methods. The popularity of qualitative methodology is on the rise in recent years. Though complementarity of quantitative and qualitative methodologies is emphasized, but it seems for the present, psychology is divided into these two camps with different epistemologies, subject matter, objectives and implications of the research.

It may be stated here that the term method in quantitative research does not have the same connotation as in qualitative research. Quantitative methods are more structured, with the step-by-step procedure laid down, which a researcher can easily learn. In qualitative research, there are no laid down steps to follow in data analysis. There is much freedom to a researcher in qualitative research to develop their own analysis procedure within a broad framework. This built-in flexibility precludes any standardization of analysis procedures, and we can only talk in terms of research methodologies (Dalal & Priya, 2015).

Quantitative Methods

These methods rely on the quantification of the psychological phenomena. Psychological phenomena are broken into distinct set of variables, quantified and subjected to further analysis. Variables are further distinguished as independent, dependent, intervening, extraneous variables and provide the basis for formulating hypotheses and theories. The quantitative data are subjected to statistical analysis to arrive at some general conclusions. The development of tests/scales, computing their reliability, validity and norms are all part of quantitative research.

This empirical–positivistic approach has dominated psychological research for more than a century and is still very much a part of the mainstream academic research. All four levels of measurement—ordinal, ranking, interval and ratio—are an integral part of such quantitative processing of data. A large number of statistical data analysis techniques have been developed—*t*-test, analysis of variance, correlation, regression analysis, factor analysis, canonical analysis and many others are available to process the data.

Qualitative Research Methods

Qualitative research often deals with lived experiences. The emphasis is on what people have gone through in terms of experiential reality. Everyday conversations, personal and social events, fears, thoughts and emotions are all subjective experiences, not objective realities. We live in a subjective world which cannot be accessed through standardized procedures, tests and tools. In order to fulfil methodological standards of objectivity, research procedures, data and findings often remain far removed from questions and concerns of everyday life.

The subjective reality which people experience and narrate is a constructed reality. It is a reconstruction of what people have gone through. They recall from their memory and reconstruct an event/experience. What we need to pay attention to is that people differ in their reporting of the same event; they differ in terms of what they pay attention to, consider important, where they fill in the missing gaps and what they consider proper to share. Furthermore, they could have a false memory, forget selectively or distort events voluntarily or involuntarily. Various qualitative methods have been developed to analyse our subjective experiences and many are still at the formative stage. Qualitative methods greatly emphasize reflectivity on the part of a researcher to introspect for own theoretical assumptions and research questions, and also one's own personal motivation and personal history which may colour their generation of data and interpretations.

The list of quantitative and qualitative methods can be endlessly large. Here some of the prominent research methods from these two categories are listed.

Quantitative Methods

Experimental methods, Qui-experiments, surveys, questionnaires, observation method, test construction and testing, field studies and so on.

Qualitative Methods

Qualitative methods are of two types:

1. **Positivistic:** Content analysis, ethnography, projective tests, case studies and archival research.

2. **Constructionist:** Grounded theory, narrative research, focus group discussion, ethno-methodology, discourse analysis, phenomenological research, conversational analysis, visual-textual analysis and so on.

Qualitative research is gaining popularity in recent years and many of these methods are still evolving. These qualitative methods primarily deal with subjective data. In positivistic qualitative data, while the effort is on quantifying subjective data, in constructionist methods, the effort is to understand the data as experiential reality. Taken together, these methods cover the whole range of possibilities in psychological research. In recent times, there has been considerable degree of epistemological and methodological plurality in the use of research methods (Metcalfe, 2005). In the mixed-method approach, both quantitative and qualitative methods are combined in a research project.

However, if one looks at what researchers really do or have done, qualitative and quantitative methods coexisted all the time (e.g., Mays & Pope, 1995) and the distinction is to a certain extent artificial (Stoppard, 2002). Academic psychology in Germany actually started with what one would today call qualitative research. But often, what persons say is not left as is, but is restructured or quantified. It involves elaborating adequate categories and scales. So, often quantification is rather the end product of data analysis that might begin qualitatively. This position is not accepted by those who hold that quantitative and qualitative data are fundamentally different and any attempt to reconcile one with the other may distort the reality. The controversy persists whether causal inferences can be drawn from qualitative data or not. Some authors in the qualitative approach think that causal explanation is inappropriate in the qualitative approach (Altwood, 2012), whereas others like Maxwell (2004) argue that causal analysis is legitimate and doable in the qualitative approach.

A Threefold Classification of Research Methodologies

Another scheme of classifying research methods is in terms of researcher–participant dichotomy. The question is on whom the research is conducted and by whom? Following the natural science model of research, psychological research is mostly conducted on the 'other person' under controlled conditions. It is only in the last 2–3 decades that psychologists have paid attention to other modes of conducting research. Taking together, the positivistic, constructionist and yoga (to be discussed in the later section) paradigms of research can be examined in terms of 'who' is the researcher. A threefold classification of research methodologies is suggested along this line. This threefold classification includes third-person, second-person and first-person research methodologies. This broader classification scheme should be appropriate to cover all possible methodologies which can be used to study health and well-being. These threefolds refer to (a) the researcher and respondent are separate, (b) both are coresearchers and (c) research on own-self. Depending on the mode of participation of the researcher in the psychology research, purpose and procedure of research will change. In psychology research, the respondent is the person selected by the researcher for data collection, according to some scheme. Most of the research methods in psychology are developed to test research hypotheses on that 'other' person. It is only in recent times that participatory research methods are being developed. Methods to conduct research on self are still at a preliminary stage of development. Research at these three levels markedly differs in their orientation, purpose, process and interpretation.

Third-person Methodologies

Psychology is primarily the study of other's behaviour and mind. The research is conducted on people selected as the research participants. Sampling procedure is used to identify the target group and then select volunteers to participate in the research from the group. Data are collected on that sample of participants, which is then processed and analysed by the researcher. In most of the psychological research, this distinction between the researcher and the subject (respondent) is maintained with role clarity and assigned responsibilities. Of course, such research can be conducted on a single respondent.

Third-person methodologies, as taken from the natural sciences, are also quite widespread in psychology. For instance, two of the main criteria of goodness in constructing psychological tests are 'objectivity' (it should not matter who conducts the test, who evaluates the test results) and 'reliability' (e.g., if the test is administered again, the similar results should be obtained). Also, all possible influences of the experimenter in psychological research are usually regarded as 'nuisance variables' and should be strictly controlled. It makes sense for examining a wide variety of psychological hypotheses, and often, the influence of extraneous variables (e.g., demographic background the experimenter and the participants) are systematically controlled.

Most of the research methods employed in academic or mainstream psychology belong to this category. It includes both quantitative and qualitative methods, where it is the other person (respondent) who is the source of data in the research.

Second-person Methodologies

In second-person, methodologies are participatory in nature in which the distinction between researcher and respondent is blurred. They work together as coresearchers in the research process to arrive at some collective solution emanating from shared experiences. It is a dynamic process of sense-making in which participants interact in the spirit of a collaborative enterprise, elicit data and even using the experimental method to answer the research questions. In second person research, the critical aspect is to build inter-subjective reality through collaborative activity so as to arrive at collective solutions. Such groups could be dyads, triads or bigger groups which interact in a research according to some plan. In health research, one needs to acknowledge that patients are not passive recipients of the treatment, but, according to a second-person approach, they do participate in the process of understanding their disease and deciding about the course of treatment, often informally; but formally also when participating for research purpose (Reddy, 2008). Such dyads could be of guru–*shishya* (teacher–disciple) or writer–reader or officer–subordinate or doctor–patient; any group of people with a common objective. People may share a common background, common interest, but still some amount of groundwork (or familiarity) is often a prerequisite to apply second-person methods.

Such participatory methods often aim to engage all stakeholders to collectively search for the solution of practical problems. As such, no distinction is made between researchers and subjects as both work together to study the problem. The focus is primarily on the experiential knowledge of action and growth. The process of research is demystified in which all seekers have an equal stake. The newly developing participatory methods (Kumar, 2002) and the Method of Cooperative Inquiry (Heron, 1996), in which participants take multiple roles as researchers and as subjects, can be effectively used to study the whole range of cultural issues in health research. Such methods are still at the developmental stage.

Second-person approaches to study consciousness are proposed by Depraz (1999) and many others. All these methods need to fulfil two conditions:

1. Providing a clear 'procedure' for accessing some phenomenal domain.
2. Providing clear means for an 'expression and validation' of the findings by a community of observers who have familiarity with procedures as mentioned in the first point.

These two conditions are relevant for other second-person methods as well. Validation of such studies can either be done by having several 'second persons' interact with the same participant, having one 'second person' interact with several participants or a combination of the two. Many of such methods have been used in anthropological and sociological research, which in recent times, are borrowed and modified to be appropriate for psychological research.

First-person Methodologies

These are pertaining to the methods employed to conduct experiments on own-self. In these studies, research is conducted to understand own physiological, psychological, paranormal and other kinds of inner experiences. Ebbinghaus was the first psychologist who conducted on himself all his memory experiments (Robinson, 1995). He prepared a learning material (mostly non-sense syllables) and subjected himself to learning of such material to know how our memory works. This kind of research, however, could not continue in psychology for long. It may be clarified here that single-subject research is not first-person research; in that research, the researcher and the subject are different persons. In a true sense, the forerunner of first-person methodologies was the introspection method. Introspection was introduced by Wilhelm Wundt in his Leipzig laboratory, where "one attends carefully to one's own sensation and reports them as objectively as possible" (as quoted in Gardner, 1987, p. 103). The subjects were required to describe the felt sensation and not the stimulus that provoke it. In a way, introspectionists were studying the elements of sensation and looking for the basic constituents of mental states. The subject matter was the mental act—such as judging, sensing, imagining or hearing—each of which reflects a sense of direction as well. Cognitive psychology continued such research in terms of thought experiment, causal attribution and imagery studies. However, it was the third-person research which dominated the field. In the area of health and well-being, first-person research was rare for almost a century. In the recent years, several empirical methodologies have been developed, which aim at "exploring the peculiarities of introspection as a cognitive process and setting up conditions under which maximal accuracy of introspective data can be ensured" (Feest, 2012, p. 12).

The first-person approach needs to ensure bracketing of personal biases and experiences—suspending judgement, a process of stepping outside of our usual, mundane and preconceived notions about how the world works, to gain greater insights and better understandings of one's mental structures and processes. Many self-reflective techniques are suggested to become aware of one's biases in such research. It was the major criticism of the introspection method of Wundt (Castellan, 2010). Another important challenge of the first-person methodologies is expression and validation of self-reported experiences. To make the first-person approach a rigorous research means that its results are shared by others, other than the respondent-researcher.

The range of relevant phenomena which can be studied is vast, including

> not only all the ordinary dimensions of human life (perception, motion, memory, imagination, speech and everyday social interactions), as well as cognitive events that can be precisely defined as tasks in laboratory experiments (for example, a protocol for visual attention), but also manifestations of mental life more fraught with meaning (dreaming, intense emotions, social tensions and altered states of consciousness). (Depraz & Gallagher, 2002, p. 2)

First-person methods concerned with the description of the "authentic and intimate contact of the subject with its own experience" may be of interest to neuroscientists, attempting to correlate brain-imaging techniques with the experience of the person. The experience of pain, for example, may be correlated with neuro-chemical changes in the brain. Such a study may be useful to therapists interested in assisting others in dealing with their ailments or in arriving at sound decision-making about the course of treatment. With the more accurate measurements of brain activity with functional magnetic resonance imagining and such other tools, neuroscientists are able to arrive at more fine-grained descriptions of experience that can be linked to neural correlates. This field of research is one of the most productive ones in the area of health and well-being (Horton & Wedding, 2008). As Nahmias (2002, p. 12) states, it might be worthwhile

> (1) to try to train subjects to attend more closely to their experiences and describe them more fully and accurately; (2) to try to develop a more precise language with which subjects can report the contents of conscious experience; and ultimately, (3) to try to map out the internal structure of conscious experience to better understand its relations to neural processes.

Accordingly, despite some reservations, it is evident that mainstream science can greatly benefit from the practical knowledge of first-person and second-person methods that have accumulated outside its traditional remit. The depth and range of the anecdotal evidence provided by many of the authors in this volume offer a number of fascinating starting points for more rigorous scientific studies. One of the challenges before health psychology is that of the first-person and second-person verification of the third-person research.

Indian Methods of Knowing

In the Indian tradition, a distinction is made between *parā vidyā* (knowledge of the self) and *aparā vidyā* (empirical knowledge) (Paranjpe, 1984). Aparā vidyā constitutes the knowledge of the social-physical world we live in and includes science and technology. This knowledge is also relevant to the problems and challenges of the world we live in. The methods of knowing in the empirical world (*pramāṇa*) are diverse and they treat mind (*mānas* or *antaḥkaranā*) as one sensory channel, which allows the understanding of pleasure and pain. Parā vidyā is the knowledge of one's higher existence, beyond the empirical world. It is the knowledge of one's higher consciousness; knowledge of that which is permanent and imperishable. Here, not only the very 'object' of knowledge is very different, but even the approach and methodology are different too (Misra, 2009). In this case, the knower is striving to know about own-self.

It is clear that academic (Western) psychology has focused only on surface reality or outer appearance. The deeper reality has escaped the attention of psychologists. Even in the study of yoga and meditation, first, the focus was only on physiological outcomes and on those psychological aspects which could be easily measured. Second, overemphasis on objectivity led to research outcomes which were trivial and dubious, contradictory and, at the best, 'obvious'. It avoided venturing into non-physical reality, mystical experiences and paranormal phenomena, which are of interest in Indian psychology. Indian psychology is spiritual and transcendental in its orientation in which the unity of spirit and matter—the union of *Puruṣa* and *Prakṛti*—comprises overall human existence. The *Puruṣa* is the supreme consciousness in each one of us, considered to be the real knower. Waking or sensory consciousness is taken as only one kind of consciousness in Indian scriptures. In contemporary psychology, it is taken as a given reality, a universal standard against which all psychological theories and knowledge are to be validated.

Different schools of thought had subscribed to different kinds of methodologies. The Charvaka school regards perception alone, the Buddhists regards perception and inference, the Sankhya and the Yoga schools regard perception, inference and testimony, the Mimamsa and the Advaita Vedantic schools regard perception, inference, comparison, testimony, presumption and non-apprehension as the sources of valid knowledge. This list can be still longer if we also include the methods listed in the other texts also. Misra (2002) has discussed some of these methods in greater detail.

Brief description of seven primary methods is given in Table 6.1.

It may be mentioned here that whereas in the Western science the emphasis is on empiricism and is considered to the best method of knowing, in Indian tradition, intuition is the most preferred and reliable method. Intuitive knowledge is the direct knowledge without any median and, therefore, uncontaminated.

Table 6.1:
Indian Methods of Knowing

1. *Pratyaksa* (empirical, perception and observation)—Objective knowledge of some object through sense organs—perception of both external and internal (bodily) objects and states through the mediation of mind.

2. *Anumāna* (inference)—Relation between what is perceived and what is deduced—knowledge derived from some other knowledge—through reasoning—both inductive and deductive reasoning.

3. *Upamāna* (comparison)—Similarity, analogy or contrast—mind draws parallels.

4. *Arthāpatti* (postulation)—Developing premises—bridging the gap in our knowledge through assumptions and suppositions.

5. *Śabda Pramāna* (verbal testimony)—Acceptance of the testimony of an authority (scriptures, specialist, expert and wise person who have attained knowledge). Accumulated knowledge through centuries of experience and experimentation. Rishis, yogis, gurus and others.

6. *Anupalabdhi* (non-cognition)—Knowledge of non-existence.

7. **Intuition**—Trans-sensory knowledge and non-mediated direct knowledge.

Yoga and Meditation as an Indian Paradigm of Research

India has a centuries-old tradition of yoga and meditation with many different systems of practices. Buddhism, Jainism, Shaiva and other schools of thought have contributed to yoga and meditational practices. Yoga is primarily considered to be a spiritual practice of attaining enlightenment and liberation (*Yoga Sutra of Patanjali*, as quoted by Swamy Satchidanand, 2008). Yoga and meditation, in the long history, have been used for improving mental and physical health, by controlling mental and bodily processes. These have been used for dealing with health problems also. Yoga and meditational techniques are now used all over the world for therapeutic purposes.

Yoga and meditation have also been used for exploration of inner experiences, as first-person methodology. As methods of research, yoga and meditation have been used for centuries to test, experiment and arrive at an experiential validation of the higher mental states. Various systems of yoga in India have developed rigorous and efficient methodology of enquiry in the domains of consciousness studies and psychology that may help us find answers to our deeper questions regarding illness, health and well-being. They can offer to modern science not only a wealth of philosophical and psychological theories of well-being, but also a rich storehouse of practical techniques to raise our individual and collective consciousness. Consciousness in the Indian context refers to the awareness one has of one's own existence (being) and its connectedness to the Supreme Being.

The purpose of yoga is to keep refining and improvising the inner instrument so that one can have a clearer understanding of the inner processes and outer reality. This is the instrument of observing (or being aware of) the higher consciousness, which is independent of waking or sensory consciousness. Sensory consciousness or the mind primarily works through sensory inputs and our accumulated memory represents the sum total of our past experiences and their fruition. Any observation and knowledge emanating from his sensory mind is bound to be biased and unreliable (Rao, 2002). It is the higher consciousness, which is independent of sensory mind, is presumed to be neutral and, as a witness, can observe mental processes and experiences. Yoga techniques are meant to clean this instrument, so that like a mirror, the higher consciousness may reflect the reality (Kapoor, 2009).

Sri Aurobindo has made a significant contribution to methodological discourse by developing intuition as a potent method of knowing. According to Sri Aurobindo, the higher consciousness of a person can grasp the essence of matter in a way which has till date escaped the physicists, who for the most part acknowledge that they have no idea what matter or energy is in itself (Sri Aurobindo, 1997).

This method, according to Sri Aurobindo, is a trans-sensory method of knowing. In the ordinary sense, we can call it knowledge through intuition and other extra-sensory means. This is a new way of knowing in which senses are not involved, Sri Aurobindo called it knowledge by identity, where we understand by being one with the object of knowing. Sri Aurobindo showed how through yoga, intuition can become a permanent state of one's being, a direct source of knowledge about the world and reality.

While concluding this discussion on Indian methods of knowing, it has to be kept in mind that though these methods have been practised for centuries to investigate consciousness, paranormal phenomena and spiritual experiences, their access is limited to serious seekers only.

They are part of an established spiritual tradition whose main objective is self-growth and development. A major challenge is to bring these methods within the ambit of scientific psychology by removing ideological overtones. For this, it is necessary that these Indian methods are critically examined within the contemporary discourse on the scientific epistemology of self-inquiry.

Yoga as a first-person methodology can be of help in bridging the gap between first-person and third-person methodologies. Yoga methods can be of help in studying subjective experiences as objective reality, which can be corroborated by an independent observer. In the studies of pain and suffering, empathic observers are found to corroborate the first-person experience. Buddhist techniques of exploration of human suffering, which have been tested and refined over 25 centuries by many generations of practitioners, provide us with invaluable leads to pursue. But mastering meditation techniques requires intensive training for several years which is impracticable for most of the health scientists. Nevertheless, methods of yoga give scientists some hope that proper methodologies can be developed for collecting the data (both first and third person), express them in suitable language and find connecting principles. We need to work on a 'fundamental theory of consciousness', that is, to unravel universal laws of the interconnected world. One problem is that yoga methodology is integral to India's spiritual tradition and how far such methodology can be reconciled with rationale theories of the west?

References

Abidi, Javed (2004). *Research study on present education scenario.* New Delhi: NPCID.

Abramson, L. Y., Seligman, M. E. P., & Teasdale, J. (1978). Learned helplessness in humans: Critique and reformulation. *Journal of Abnormal Psychology, 87,* 49–74.

Acton, N. (1983). Address by the Secretary General, Rehabilitation International. In O. Shirley (Ed.), *A cry for health: Poverty and disability in the Third World.* New York: The Third World Group for Disabled People.

Adair, J. (2006). Creating indigenous psychologies: Insights from empirical social studies of the science of psychology. In U. Kim, K. S. Yang & K. K. Hwang (Eds.), *Indigenous and cultural psychology: Understanding people in context* (pp. 467–485). New York, NY: Springer.

Adler, R. (2009). Engel's Biopsychosocial Model is still Relevant Today. *Journal of Psychosomatic Research, 67,* 607–611.

Agarwal, M., & Dalal, A. K. (1993). Beliefs about the world and recovery from myocardial infarction. *Journal of Social Psychology, 133,* 385–394.

Agarwal, M., & Naidu, R. K. (1988). Impact of desirable and undesirable life events on health. *Journal of Personality and Clinical Studies, 4,* 53–62.

Agrawal, M., Dalal, A. K., Agrawal, R. K., & Agrawal, D. K. (1994). Positive life orientation and psychological recovery of myocardial infraction patients. *Social Science and Medicine, 38,* 25–130.

Ajzen, I., & Fishbein, M. (1980). *Understanding attitudes and predicting social behavior.* Englewood Cliff, NJ: Prentice Hall.

Altwood, C. M. (2012). The distinction between qualitative and quantitative research methods is problematic. *Qualitative Research, 46,* 1417–1429.

American Hospital Association. (2008). Press release. Retrieved from http://www.aha.org/aha/press-release/2008/080915-pr-cam.html on 18 November 2010.

Anand, J. (2006). Toward a conceptual formulation of psychological healing. *Psychological Studies, 51*(2), 119–126.

———. (2011). *Healing narratives of women: A psychological perspective.* Jaipur: Rawat.

Anand, J., & Dalal, A. K. (2013). Concept, characteristics and process of psychological healing. In G. Misra (Ed.), *History of science, philosophy and culture: Psychology and psychoanalysis* (Vol. 9, pp. 693–710). New Delhi: Pratyush Publications.

Armstrong, D. (1987). Theoretical tension in biopsychosocial medicine. *Social Science and Medicine, 25,* 1213–1218.

ASSOCHAM Report. (2011). *Access to health care report.* New Delhi: The Associated Chambers of Commerce & Industry of India.

Bajpai, N., & Goyal, S. (2004). *Primary health care in India: Coverage and quality. Working paper no. 15.* New York: Earth Institute, Columbia University.

Bakheit, A., & Shanmugalingam, V. (1997). A study of the attitudes of a rural Indian community towards people with disability. *Clinical Rehabilitation, 11*(4), 329–334.

Banerjee, M. (2000). *Whither indigenous medicine.* Retrieved from http://www.indiaseminar.com/2000/489.html on 19 August 2012.

Banerji, D. (2003). *Primary health care in India: An overview.* Guest Lecture at the National Seminar on Health for All in the New Millennium, NIHFW, New Delhi, February 24–26.

Baum, A., & Posluszny, D. M. (1999). Health psychology: Mapping bio-behavioral contributions to health and illness. *Annual Review of Psychology, 50,* 137–163.

Becker, M. H., & Maiman, L. A. (1975). Sociobehavioural determinants of compliance with health and medical care recommendations. *Medical Care, 13,* 10–24.

Benson, H. (1997). *Timeless healing: The power and biology of beliefs.* New York: Sribner.

Berger, P. L., & Luckmann, T. (1966). *The social construction of reality. A treatise in the sociology of knowledge.* Harmondsworth: Penguin Books.

Berman, V. M., Dalal, A. K., & Anthony, L. (1984). Connotation of handicapped label in India. *Psychologia, 27,* 115–121.

Berry, J. W. (1989). Imposed etics-emics-derived etics: Operationalization of a compelling idea. *International Journal of Psychology, 24,* 721–735.

———. (2000). Cross-cultural psychology: A symbiosis of culture and comparative approaches. *Asian Journal of Social Psychology, 3,* 197–205.

Bhasin, V. (2007). *Medical anthropology: A review.* Delhi: Department of Anthropology, University of Delhi.

Bhattacharyya, D. (2001). Effect of type A behaviour and locus of control in the coping styles: A study on coronary heart patients. *Indian Journal of Clinical Psychology, 28*(2), 181–185.

Bhugra, B., & Bhui, K. (2007). *Textbook of cultural psychiatry.* Cambridge: Cambridge University Press.

Birbeck, G. (2000). Barriers to care for patients with neurologic disease in rural Zambia. *Archives of Neurology, 57*(March), 43–49.

———. (2004). *Traditional health systems and national policy.* Retrieved from http://users.ox.ac.uk/~gree0179/C on 19 August 2012.

Bonanno, G. A. (2004). Loss, trauma, and human resilience: Have we underestimated the human capacity to thrive after extremely aversive events? *American Psychologist, 59,* 20–28.

Burne, J. (2002, June 20). Make-believe medicine. *The Guardian.* Retrieved from http://www.guardian.co.uk/Archive/Article/0,4273,4444420,00.html on 1 February 2013.

Capra, F. (1983). *The turning point.* Glasgow: Flamingo.

Cassell, E. J. (1991). *The nature of suffering and the goals of medicine.* Oxford, UK: Oxford University Press.

Cassileth, B. R. (1998*). The alternative medicine handbook: The complete reference guide to alternative and complementary therapies.* New York: W. W. Norton.

Castellan, C. M. (2010). Quantitative and qualitative research: A view for clarity. *International Journal of Education*, *2*(2), 242–253.

Charak (1962). *Charaka Samhita* (K. N. Pandey, & G. N. Chaturevedi, Trans.). Varanasi: Chowkhambha Vidya Bhavan.

Chatterjee, M. (1993). Health for too many: India's experiments with truth. In J. Rohde, M. Chatterjee & D. Morley (Eds.), *Reaching health for all*. New Delhi: Oxford University Press.

Chattopadhyaya, D. (1982). Case for a critical analysis of the *Charaka Samhita*. In D. Chattopadhyaya (Ed.), *Studies in the History of Science in India* (Vol. 1). New Delhi: Centre for the Studies in Civilizations.

Chopra, D. (1990). *Quantum healing: Exploring the frontiers of mind–body medicine*. New York: Bantam Books.

Chaudhury, N., Hammer, J., Kremer, M., Muralidharan, K., & Rogers, F. H. (2006). Missing in action: teacher and health worker absence in developing countries. *The Journal of Economic Perspectives*, *20*, 91–116.

Cobb, S. (1976). Social support as a moderator of life stress. *Psychosomatic Medicine*, *38*, 300–314.

Cohen, F., & Lazarus, R. S. (1979). Coping with the stresses of illness. In G. C. Stone, F. Cohen & N. E. Adler (Eds.), *Health psychology: A handbook*. San Francisco: Jossey-Bass.

Confederation of Indian Industry. (2010). *India health report*. New Delhi: The Confederation of Indian Industry.

Conrad, P. (1994). Wellness as virtue: Morality and the pursuit of health. *Culture, Medicine and Psychiatry*, *18*, 385–401.

Cousins, N. (1979). *Anatomy of an illness*. New York: Norton.

Crocker, J., Cornwell, B., & Major, B. (1993). The stigma of overweight: Affective consequences of attributional ambiguity. *Journal of Personality and Social Psychology*, *64*, 60–70.

CSIE. (2004). *Inclusive education: Disabled person and education in the new UN disability convention*. Retrieved from www.csie.org.uk on 8 August 2013.

Dalal, A. K. (1988). Reactions to tragic life events: An attributional model of psychological recovery. In A.K. Dalal (Ed.), *Attribution theory and research*. New Delhi: Wiley Eastern.

———. (1991). A matter of faith. *Times of India: Sunday Edition* (October 11). New Delhi.

———. (1999). Health beliefs and coping with a chronic illness. In G. Misra (Ed.), *Psychological perspectives in stress and health*. New Delhi: Concept.

———. (2000a). Living with a chronic disease: Healing and psychological adjustment in Indian society. *Psychology and Developing Societies*, *12*(1), 67–82.

———. (2000b). Social attitudes and rehabilitation of people with disability: The Indian experience. *Arab Journal of Rehabilitation*, *5*, 15–21.

———. (2001). Health psychology. In J. Pandey (Ed.), *Psychology in India Revisited* (Vol. 1, pp. 356–411). New Delhi: SAGE Publications.

———. (2006). Social interventions to moderate discriminatory attitudes: The case of the physically challenged in India. *Psychology, Health & Medicine*, *11*(3), 374–382.

Dalal, A. K. (2010). Psychosocial interventions for community development. In G. Misra (Ed.), *Psychology in India* (Vol. 3). New Delhi: Pearson.

———. (2011). Folk wisdom and traditional healing practices: Some lessons for modern psychotherapies. In M. Cornelissen, G. Misra & S. Verma (Eds.), *Foundations of Indian psychology* (pp. 21–35). New Delhi: Pearson.

———. (2013). Salience of indigenous healing practices for health care programmes in India. In R. C. Tripathi & Sinha, Y. (Eds.), *Psychology as a policy science* (pp. 193–210). New Delhi: Springer.

———. (2015). *Health beliefs and coping with chronic diseases*. New Delhi: SAGE Publications.

Dalal, A. K. & Misra, G. (2011). *New direction in health psychology*. New Delhi: SAGE Publications.

Dalal, A. K., & Pande, N. (1995). A community intervention programme for changing attitude toward disability. *The Social Engineer, 4*, 16–25.

Dalal, A. K., & Priya, R. (2015). Introduction to qualitative research. In R. Priya and A. K. Dalal (Eds.), *Qualitative research on well-being and self-growth: Contemporary Indian perspectives*. New Delhi: Routledge.

Dalal, A. K., & Ray, S. (2005). Social dimension of health and well-being: An overview of research trends. In A. K. Dalal & S. Ray (Eds.), *Social dimensions of health*. Jaipur: Rawat.

Dalal, A. K., Kumar, S., & Gokhale, D. (2000). *Participatory evaluation of community based rehabilitation*. Project report presented to Department of Psychology, University of Allahabad, Allahabad.

Dalal, A. K., Pande, N., Dhawan, N., Dwijendra, D., & Berry, J. (2000). *The mind matters: Disability attitudes and community rehabilitation*. Allahabad, India: University of Allahabad.

de Haan, A. (1997). *Poverty and social exclusion: A comparison of debates on deprivation. Working Paper* 2, Poverty Research Unit, Sussex University, Brighton.

Denollet, J. (2000). Type D personality: A potential factor redefined. *Journal of Psychosomatic Research, 49*(4), 255–266.

———. (2004). Type D personality in perspective. *Journal of Psychosomatic Research, 56*, 584–596.

Denzin, N. K., & Lincoln, Y. S. (2005). *The Sage handbook of qualitative research* (3rd Edition). London: SAGE Publications.

Department of Rural Development. (1985). *Report on the committee to review the existing administrative arrangements for rural development and poverty alleviation programmes (CAARD)*. New Delhi: Ministry of Agriculture, Government of India.

Depraz, N. (1999). The phenomenological reduction as praxis. In F. J. Varela, and J. Shear (Ed.), *The view from within*. Exeter: Imprint Academic.

Depraz, N., & Gallagher, S. (2002). Phenomenology and the cognitive sciences: Editorial introduction. *Phenomenology and the Cognitive Sciences, 1*(1), 1–6.

Devi, M. (2002). *The book of the hunter* (Sagaree, & M. Sengupta, Trans.). New Delhi: Seagull Books.

Diaz, J. L. (1997). A patterned process approach to brain, consciousness and behavior. *Philosophical Psychology, 10*, 179–195.

Diener, E. (1984). Subjective well-being. *Psychological Bulletin, 95*, 542–575.

Diener, E. (2000). Subjective well-being: The science of happiness, and a proposal for a national index. *American Psychologist, 55*, 34–43.

Diener, E., & Biswas-Diener, R. (2008). *Happiness: Unlocking the mysteries of psychological wealth.* New York: Wiley-Blackwell.

Diener, E., Oishi, S., & Lucas, R. E. (2003). Personality, culture, and subjective well-being: Emotional and cognitive evaluations of life. *Annual Review of Psychology, 54*, 403–425.

Dilthey, W. (1996). *Hermeneutics and the study of history (Vol. 4).* Princeton, NJ: Princeton University Press.

Directorate of Town Panchayats. (2008). *Activities of empowerment.* Chennai: Directorate of Town Panchayats.

Draft Proposal. (2015). *National health policy.* New Delhi: Ministry of Health and Family Welfare.

Draft Report. (2013). *13th Five Year Plan.* New Delhi: Planning Commission.

———. (2014). *Indian health care sector report.* New Delhi: Ministry of Health and Family Welfare.

Dreze, J., & Sen, A. (2002). *India: Development and participation.* New Delhi: Oxford University Press.

DSM-4-TR. (2004). *Diagnostic statistical manual.* Washington: American Psychological Association.

DSM-5. (2013). *Diagnostic statistical manual.* Washington: American Psychological Association.

Dube, S. C. (1990). *Tradition and development.* New Delhi: Vikas Publishing House.

Dunbar, F. (1943). *Psychosomatic diagnosis.* New York: Hoeber.

EFA Global Monitoring Report. (2008). *Education for all by 2015: Will we make it?* Geneva: UNESCO.

Ellich, E. (1974). *Medical nemesis.* London: Calder & Boyars.

Elwan, A. (1999). *Poverty and disability: A review of the literature.* Background Paper for the World Development Report 2000/2001. Washington, D.C.: World Bank.

Engel, G. L. (1977). The need for a new medical model: A challenge for biomedicine. *Science, 196*, 129–136.

Erwin, N. (1959). Self-healing is a mechanism prevalent worldwide. *Journal of Tropical Diseases, 42*, 150–158.

ESCAP. (1993). *Asia and Pacific decade of disabled persons, 1993–2002: The starting point.* New York: United Nations.

Esses, V. M., & Beaufoy, S. L. (1994). Determinants of attitudes towards people with disabilities. *Journal of Social Behaviour and Personality, 9*, 43–64.

Eyben, R., & Ferguson, C. (2000). *Realizing human rights for poor people: Strategies for achieving the international development targets.* London: Department for International Aid.

Eysenck, H. J. (1988). Personality, stress and cancer: prediction and prophylaxis. *British Journal of Medical Psychology, 61*(Pt. 1), 57–75.

Feagin, J. R. (1972). Poverty: We still believe that God helps those who help themselves. *Psychology Today, 6*(6), 101–129.

Feather, N. T. (1974). Explanations of poverty in Australian and American samples: The person, society, or fate? *Australian Journal of Psychology, 26*(3), 199–216.

Feest, U. (2012). Introspection as a method and introspection as a feature of consciousness. *Inquiry, 55*(1), 1–16.

Fields, G. P. (2001). *Religious therapeutics: Body and health in yoga, Āyurveda and tantra.* New York: State University of New York.

Fine, M., & Asch, A. (1988). Disability beyond stigma: Social interaction, discrimination, and activism. *Journal of Social Issues, 44,* 3–22.

Finlay, L. (2009). Debating phenomenological research methods. *Phenomenology and Practice, 3*(1), 6–65.

Frank, J. D. (1975). The faith that heals. *Johns Hopkins Medical Journal, 137,* 127–131.

Frank, J. D., & Frank, J. B. (1991). *Persuasion and healing.* London: The John Hopkins University Press.

Fredrickson, B. L. (2001). The role of positive emotions in positive psychology: The broaden-and-build theory of positive emotions. *American Psychologist, 56,* 218–226.

Gallacher, J. E. J., Sweetnam, P. M., Yarnell, J. W. G., Elwood, P. C., & Stansfeld, S. A. (2003). Is type A really a trigger for coronary heart disease events? *Psychosomatic Medicine, 65,* 339–346.

Gardner, H. (1987). *The mind's new science.* New York: Basic Book.

Gergen, K. J. (1982). *The transformation of social knowledge.* New York: Springer Verlag.

———. (1985). The social constructionist movement in modern psychology. *American Psychologist, 40,* 266–275.

———. (1988). *The saturated self.* New York: Basic Books

———. (1994). *Realities and relationships.* Cambridge Mass: Harvard University Press.

Ghai, A. (2001). Marginalisation and disability: Experiences from the Third World. In M. Priestley (Ed.), *Disability and the life course: Global perspectives* (pp. 26–37). Cambridge: Cambridge University Press.

———. (2010). The psychology of disabled people. In G. Misra (Ed.), *Psychology in India* (Vol. 3). New Delhi: Pearson.

Gielen, U. P., Fish, J. M., & Draguns, J. G. (2004). *Handbook of culture, therapy and healing.* London: Lawrence Erlbaum.

Giorgi, A. (1995). Phenomenological psychology. In J. A. Smith, R. Harré & K. van Langenhove (Eds.), *Rethinking psychology.* London: SAGE Publications.

Giri, A. K. (1998). *Global transformation: Postmodernity and beyond.* Jaipur: Rawat Publications.

Glass, D. C. (1976). *Behavior patterns, stress and coronary disease.* Hillsdale, NJ: Earlbaum.

Glasser, W. (1976). *Positive addiction.* New York: Harper & Row.

Goffman, E. (1963). *Stigma: Notes on the management of spoiled identity.* Englewood Cliffs, NJ: Prentice Hall.

Goldberg, A. (1994). Farewell to the objective analyst. *International Journal of Psychoanalysis, 75*(21), 23–30.

Government of India. (2007). *Report on conditions of work and promotion of livelihoods in the unorganised sector.* Report presented to National Commission for Enterprises in the Unorganised Sector, August.

Groce, N. (1990). Traditional folk belief systems and disabilities: An important factor in policy planning. *One in Ten, 8,* 1–4.

Gower, B. (1997). *Scientific methods: A historical and philosophical introduction.* New York: Routledge.

Gupta, B. (1998). Indigenous medicine in nineteenth and twentieth century Bengal. In C. Leslie (Ed.), *Asian medical systems: A contemporary study* (pp. 368–378). Delhi: Motilal Banarasidass.

Gupta, U, Shama, G. K., Narayan, R., & Gupta, B. S. (2002). Perceived social support in relation to stress, anxiety and depression in coronary heart disease. *Indian Journal of Clinical Psychology, 29*(1), 27–34.

Gurung, R. A. R. (2014). *Health psychology: A cultural approach.* Belmont, CA: Cengage Learning.

Harihar, S. (2012). Use and overuse of antibiotics in primary health care. *Indian Journal of Psychosomatic Medicine, 14,* 24–28.

Harriss-White, B. (1996). *The political economy of disability and development, with special reference to India.* UNRISD Discussion Paper. Geneva: United Nations Research Institute for Social Development.

Hatfield, G. (2005). Introspective evidence in psychology. In P. Achinstein (Ed.), *Scientific evidence: Philosophical theories and applications* (p. XXX). Baltimore, MD: Johns Hopkins University Press.

Hegarty, S. (1995). *Review of the present situation in special needs education.* Paris: UNESCO.

Heron, J. (1996). *Cooperative inquiry: Research into the human condition.* London: SAGE Publications.

Heumann, J. (2012). *Special advisor's remarks on inclusive development.* New York: The Office of Policy Planning and Public Diplomacy. Retrieved from http://www.humanrights.gov/tag/judith-heumann/ on 8 August 2013.

Hewson, M. G. (1998). Traditional healers in Southern Africa. *Annals of International Medicine, 128*(12), 1029–1034.

Hewstone, M. (1994). Revision and change of stereotypic beliefs: In search of the sub-typing model. In S. Stroebe & M. Hewstone (Eds.), *European Review of Social Psychology* (Vol. 5). Chichester: Wiley.

Hoogeveen, J. (2005). Measuring welfare for small but vulnerable groups: Poverty and disability in Uganda. *Journal of African Economies, 14*(4), 603–631.

Horton, A. M., & Wedding, D. (2008). *Handbook of neuropsychology.* London: Springer.

Hulme, D., Moore, K., & Shepherd, A. (2001). *Chronic poverty: Meanings and analytical frameworks.* Chronic Poverty Research Centre Working Paper 2. Institute of Development Policy and Management/CPRC, Manchester.

Husserl, E. (1989). *Ideas pertaining to a pure phenomenological philosophy. Second book: Studies in the phenomenology of constitution.* The Hague: Kluwer Academic Publishers.

ILO, UNESCO, & WHO. (2004). *CBR: A strategy for rehabilitation, equalization of opportunities, poverty reduction and social inclusion of people with disabilities.* Joint position paper. Geneva: WHO, ILO, and UNESCO.

ILO. (2002). *Disability and poverty reduction strategies: How to ensure that access of persons with disabilities to decent and productive work is part of the PRSP process.* Geneva: International Labour Office.

———. (2003). *Time for equality in work.* Geneva: ILO.

Jacoby, A. (1994). Felt versus enacted stigma: A concept revisited. *Social Science and Medicine, 38*, 269–274.

Jain, L. C., Krishnamurthi, B. V. & Tripathi, P. M. (1985). *Grass without roots: Rural development programmes under government auspices.* New Delhi: SAGE Publications.

James, W. (1890). *Principles of psychology.* New York: H. Holt and Company.

Janis, I. L. (1958). *Psychological stress.* New York: Wiley.

Jayasunder, R. (2012). Contrasting approach to health and disease: Āyurveda and bio-medicine. In V. Sujata & L. Abraham (Eds.), *Medicine, state and society: Indigenous medicine and medical pluralism in contemporary India* (pp. 37–58). New Delhi: Orient Blackswan.

Kakar, S. (1982). *Shamans, mystics and doctors.* New Delhi: Oxford University Press.

———. (1991). *The analyst and the mystic.* New Delhi: Viking.

———. (2003). Psychoanalysis and Eastern spiritual healing traditions. *Journal of Analytical Psychology, 48*(5), 659–678.

———. (2008a). *Mad and divine: Spirit and psyche in the modern world.* Delhi: Oxford University Press.

———. (2008b). *Culture and psyche: The selected essays.* Delhi: Oxford University Press.

———. (2009). *India analysed: Sudhir Kakar in conversation with Ramin Jahanbegloo.* Delhi: Oxford University Press.

Kapoor, R. L. (2003). *What is psychotherapy?* Unpublished report, National Institute of Advanced Studies, Bangalore.

———. (2009). *Another way to live.* New Delhi: Penguin Books India.

Kazarian, S., & Evans, D. (2001). Health psychology and culture: Embracing the 21st Century. In S. Kazarian and D. Evans (Eds.), *Handbook of cultural health psychology.* Waltham: Academic Press.

Keyes, C. L. (1988). Social well-being. *Social Psychology Quarterly, 62*, 121–140.

Kiecolt-Glaser, J. K., Fisher, L. D., Ogrock, P., Stout, J. C., Speicher, C. E., & Glaser, R. (1997). Marital quality, marital disruption and immune function. *Psychosomatic Medicine, 9*, 13–34.

Kiecolt-Glaser, J. K., Garner, W., Speicher, C. E., Penn, G. M., Holliday, J., & Glaser, R. (1984). Psychosocial modifiers of immunocompetence in medical students. *Psychosomatic Medicine, 46*, 7–14.

Kitayama, S., & Cohen, D. (2007). *Handbook of cultural psychology.* New York: Guilford.

Kleinman, A. (1980). *Patients and healers in the contexts of culture.* California: University of California Press.

———. (1987). *The illness narratives: Suffering, healing, and the human condition.* New York: Basic Books.

———. (1988). *The illness narratives.* New York: Basic Books.

Koenig, H. G. (1999). *The healing power of faith: Science explores medicine's last great frontier.* New York, NY: Simon & Schuster.

Kothari, M. L., & Mehta, L. (1988). Violence in modern medicine. In A. Nandy (Ed.), *Science, hegemony ad violence.* New Delhi: Oxford University Press.

Krishnakumar, A. (2004, November 20–December 3). An unhealthy trend. *Frontline, 21*(24), 18–19.

Kubzansky, L. D., Sparrow, D., Vokonas, P., & Kawachi, I. (2001). Is the glass half empty or half full? A prospective study of optimism and coronary heart disease in the normative aging study. *Psychosomatic Medicine, 63,* 910–916.

Kuhn, T. S. (1970). *The structure of scientific revolutions* (2nd Edition). Chicago: University of Chicago Press.

———. (2002). *Methods for community development.* New Delhi: SAGE Publications.

Kuppuswami, B. (1977). *Dharma and society.* New Delhi: Macmillan.

Lang, R. (1998). Guest editorial: A critique of the disability movement. *Asia Pacific Disability Rehabilitation Journal, 9*(1), 1–12.

Lazarus, R. S. (1966). *Psychological stress and the coping process.* New York: McGraw Hill.

———. (1983). The costs and benefits of denial. In S. Bresnitz (Ed), *Denial of stress* (pp. 1–30). Madison, CT: International Universities Press.

———. (1984). On the primacy of cognition. *American Psychologist, 39,* 124–129.

Lazarus, R. S., & Folkman, S. (1984). *Stress, appraisal and coping.* New York: Springer.

Lee, H. (1999). *Discussion paper for Oxfam: Disability as a development issue and how to integrate a disability perspective into the SCO.* Oxford: Oxfam Publishing.

Lele, R. D. (1986). Āyurveda and modern medicine. Mumbai: Bharatiya Vidya Bhawan.

Leslie, C. (1998). *Asian medical systems: A comparative study.* Varanasi Motilal Banarasidas.

Levine, J. (2008). How faith heals: A theoretical model. *Explore, 5,* 77–96.

Lo, H. T., & Fung, K. (2003). Culturally competent psychotherapy. *Canadian Journal of Psychiatry, 48,* 161–170.

Lwanga-Ntale, C. (2003). *Chronic poverty and disability in Uganda.* Chronic Poverty Research Centre Working Paper. Institute of Development Policy and Management/ CPRC, Manchester.

Mallory, B. L. (1993). Changing beliefs about disability in developing countries: Historical factors and sociocultural variables. In B. L. Mallory, R. W. Nichols, J. I. Charlton & K. Marfo (Eds.), *Traditional and changing views of disability in developing societies: Causes, consequences, cautions.* Durham, NH: International Exchange of Experts and Information in Rehabilitation.

Manohar, R. (2013). Concept of health in Āyurveda. In A. Morandi, & A. N. N. Nabmi (Ed.), *An integrated view of health and well-being: Bridging Indian and western knowledge.* New York: Springer.

Marriott, M. (1955). *Village India: Studies in the little community.* Chicago: University of Chicago Press.

Marks, D. F. (2002). *The health psychology reader.* London: SAGE Publications.

Mason, J. W. (1971). A re-evaluation of the concept of 'non-specificity' in stress theory. *Journal of Psychiatric Research, 8,* 323–333.

Mather, M. (2009). *Children in immigrant families chart new path.* Washington, D.C.: Population Reference Bureau. Retrieved from http://www.prb.org/pdf09/immigrantchildren.pdf on 16 September 2015.

Maxwell, J. A. (2004). Causal explanation, qualitative research, and scientific inquiry in education. *Educational Research, 33*(2), 3–11.

Mays, N., & Pope, C. (1995). Rigour and qualitative research. *British Medical Journal, 311,* 109–112.

McGregor, S. L. T., & Murnane, J. A. (2010). Paradigm, methodology and method: Intellectual integrity in consumer scholarship. *International Journal of Consumer Studies, 34*(4), 419–427.

McRobert, G. R. (1929). William Harvey's message to India. *The Indian Medical Gazette,* April, 225–228.

Mechanic, D., & Schlesinger, M. (1996). The impact of managed care on patients' trust in medical care and their physicians. *Journal of American Medical Association, 275*(21), 1693–1697

Metcalfe, M. (2005). Generalizations: Learning across epistemological forum. *Qualitative Social Science, 6*(1), 29–38.

Miles, M. (1996). Community, individual or information development? Dilemmas of concept and culture in South Asian disability planning. *Disability and Society, 11*(4), 485–500.

———. (2000). Disability in south Asia: From millennium to millennium. *Asia Pacific Disability Rehabilitation Journal, 11*(1), 9–12.

Miller, F. G., Colloca, L., & Kaptchuk, T. J. (2009). The placebo effect: Illness and interpersonal healing. *Perspectives in Biology and Medicine, 52*(4), 518–524.

Miller, J. G. (1997). Theoretical issues in cultural psychology and social construction. In J. W. Berry, Y. Poortinga & J. Pandey (Eds.), *Handbook of cross-cultural psychology: Theoretical and methodological perspectives* (Vol. 1). Boston: Allyn & Bacon.

Miltiades, H. B. (2002). The social and psychological effect of an adult child's emigration on nonimmigrant Asian Indian elderly parents. *Journal of Cross Cultural Gerontology, 17,* 33–55.

———. (1948). *Report of the committee on indigenous systems of medicine,* Chairman Sir R.N. Chopra, New Delhi.

Ministry of Health. (1946). *Report of the health survey committee,* Chairman Sir R.N. Bhore, New Delhi.

Misra, G. (2002). Knowing in the Indian tradition. In G. Misra & A. Mohanty (Eds.), *Perspectives on indigenous psychology.* New Delhi: Concept.

Misra, G., & Mohanty, A. (2002). *Perspectives on indigenous psychology.* New Delhi: Concept.

Misra, L. C. (2004). *Scientific basis for Āyurvedic therapies.* Boca Raton, Florida: CRC Press.

Misra, V. N. (2009). *The structure of Indian mind.* New Delhi: Lal Bahudar Shastri Rashtriya Sanskrit Vidyapeeth.

Moerman, D., Jonas, W., Bush, P., Edwards, R., Herxheimer, A., Kleijnen, J., Roberts, A., Schlitz, M., Solfvin, J., van der Geest, S., & Watkins, A. (1996). Placebo effects and research in alternative and conventional medicine. *Clinical Journal Integrated Traditional Western Medicine, 2,* 141–148.

Mohanty, J. N. (1988). Phenomenology and Indian philosophy: The concept of rationality. *Journal of the British Society for phenomenology, 19*(3), 269–270.

Mohanty, A., & Misra, G. (2000). Introduction. In A. K. Mohanty & G. Misra (Eds.), *Psychology of poverty and disadvantage.* New Delhi: Concept.

Mondal, P. (1996). Psychiatry in ancient India: Toward an alternative standpoint. *NIMHANS Journal, 14*(3), 166–199.

Moore, T. (1998). *Prescription for disaster.* New York: Dell Publishing.

Muggeridge, M. (1997, September 9). In a 1968 BBC interview: Being unwanted is the worst disease. *Daily Telegraph, p.* 17.

Myrdal, G. (1944). *An American dilemma: The Negro problem and modern democracy.* New York: Harper Press.

Nahmias, E. A. (2002). Verbal reports on contents of consciousness. *Psyche,* 8(21), 1436–1441.

Nanda, M. (2009). *The God market: How globalization is making India more Hindu.* New Delhi: Random House.

National Medical Statistics. (2013). *National health statistics of 2012.* New Delhi: National Institute of Medical Statistics.

National Sample Survey Organisation. (2004). *Prevalence of disability in India.* New Delhi: National Sample Survey Organisation.

NCEUS. (2007). *Report on conditions of work and promotion of livelihoods in the unorganised sector.* New Delhi: National Commission for Enterprises in the Unorganized Sector.

O'Hara, M. (2000). Emancipatory therapeutic practices for a new era: A work of retrieval. In Kirk J. Schneider, James F. T. Bugantal & J. F. Pierson (Eds.), *Handbook of Humanistic Psychology.* London: SAGE Publications.

Osler, W. (1910, June 18). The faith that heals. *British Medical Journal, 1*(1258), 1470–1472.

Pant, P., & Bagrodia, P. (2003). A comparative study of male and female drug addicts and various psychological factors. *Social Science International, 19,* 65–72.

Pant, S. K., & Pandey, J. (2004). *Social development in rural India.* Jaipur: Rawat Publications.

Papakostas, Y. G., & Christodoulou, G. (2010). Cognitive psychotherapy and the placebo effect. *European Psychiatric Review, 3*(1), 13–15.

Paranjpe, A. C. (1984). *Theoretical psychology: The meeting of East and West.* New York: Plenum Press.

Parnas, J., Sass, L. A., & Zahavi, D. (2013). Rediscovering psychopathology: The epistemology and phenomenology of the psychiatric object. *Schizophrenia Bulletin, 39*(2), 270–277.

Pederson, S. S., Ong, A. T. L., Sonnenschein, K. Serruys, P. W., Erdman, R. A. M., & van Domburg, R. T. (2006). Type D personality and diabetes predict the onset of depressive symptoms in patients after percutaneous coronary intervention. *American Heart Journal, 151*(2), e1-367.e6.

Peterson, C., Seligman, M. E. P., & Vaillant, G. E. (1988). Pessimistic explanatory style in a risk factor for physical illness: A thirty-five year longitudinal study. *Journal of Personality and Social Psychology, 55,* 23–27.

Planning Commission of India. (1952). First five year plan (1952–1957). New Delhi: Government of India.

———. (1992). *Fifth five year plan (1992–1997).* New Delhi: Government of India.

———. (2001). *Approach paper to the tenth five year plan (2002–2007).* New Delhi: Government of India.

———. (2004). *Tenth Five Year Plan (2002–2007).* New Delhi: Government of India.

Porter, R. (2002). *Blood and guts: A short history of medicine.* New York: W. W. Norton and Company.

Prabhu P. N. (1963). *Hindu social organizations.* Bombay: Popular Prakashan.

Price, J. M., & Pecjak, V. (2003). Obesity and stigma: Important issues in women's health. *Psychology Science, 45* (Supplement II), 6–42.

Project Report. (2014). *ACCESS primary healthcare research project.* New Delhi: ACCESS International.

Qadeer, I. (2001). Debt payment and devaluating elements of public health. *Economic and Political Weekly, 37*(1), 12–16.

Radhakrishnan S. (1926). *The Hindu view of life.* Bombay: Blakie.

Radhakrishnan, R., Rao, K. H., Ravi, C., & Reddy, B. S. (2006). Chronic poverty and malnutrition in India: Incidence and determinants. In A. K. Mehta & A. Shepherd (Eds.), *Chronic Poverty and Development Policy.* New Delhi: SAGE Publications.

Radley, A. (1994). *Making sense of an illness.* London: SAGE Publications.

Raina, B. L. (1990). *Health sciences in ancient India.* New Delhi: Commonwealth Publishers.

Rao, K. R. (2002). *Consciousness studies: Cross-cultural perspective.* Jefferson, NC: McFerland.

Rasmussen, H. N., Scheier, M. F., & Greenhouse, J. B. (2009). Optimism and physical health: A meta-analytic review. *Annals of Behavioral Medicine, 37*, 239–256.

Ricoeur, P. (1970). *Freud and philosophy: An essay on interpretation* (D. Savage, Trans.). New Haven: Yale University Press.

Reddy, V. (2008). *How infants know minds.* Cambridge, MA: Harvard University Press.

Robinson, D. N. (1995). *An intellectual history of psychology.* Madisone, WC: University of Wisconsin Press.

Rosenman, R. H., Brand, R. J., Sholtz, R. I., & Friedman, M. (1976). Multivariate prediction of coronary heart disease during 8.5 year follow-up in the Western Collaborative Group Study. *The American Journal of Cardiology, 37(6)*, 903–910.

Rosenstock, I. M. (1974). Historical origins of the health belief model. *Health Education Monographs, 2*, 328–335.

Rosenthal, R. (1976). *Experimenter effects in behavioral research.* NY: Appleton-Century-Crofts.

Royle, J. F. (1837). *An Essay on the antiquity of Hindoo medicine.* London: Allen & Co.

Ryan, R. M., & Deci, E. L. (2001). On happiness and human potentials: A review of research on hedonic and eudiamonic well-being. *Annual Review of Psychology, 52*, 141–166.

Salagame, K. K. K. (2013). Perspectives on reality in Indian tradition and their implication for health and well-being. In A. Morandi & A. N. N. Nabmi (Eds.), *An integrated view of health and well-being: Bridging Indian and western knowledge.* New York: Springer.

Saligman, M. E. P. (2008). Positive psychology. *Applied Psychology, 57* (issue supplement: Health & Well-being), 3–18.

Salzano, R. (2003). Taming stress. *Scientific American, 289*, 88–98.

Saracci, R. (1997). The World Health Organization needs to reconsider its definition of Health. *Bulletin of Medical Journal, 314*, 1409–1410.

Sartorius, N. (2002). *Fighting for mental health.* Cambridge, UK: Cambridge University Press.

Sayce, L. (1998). Stigma, discrimination and social exclusion: What's in a word? *Journal of Mental Health, 7,* 331–343.

Scheier, M. F., & Carver, C. S. (1985). Optimism, coping and health: Assessment and implications of generalized outcome expectancies. *Health Psychology, 4,* 219–247.

Scheier, M. F., Weintraub, J. K., & Carver, C. S. (1986). Divergent strategies of optimists and pessimists. *Journal of Personality and Social Psychology, 51,* 1257–1264.

Schleifer, S. J., Eckholdt, H. M., Cohen, J., & Keller, S. E. (1993). Analysis of partial variance (APV) as a statistical approach to control day to day variation in immune assays. *Brain Behavior Immunology, 7,* 243–252.

Schleifer, S. J., Keller, S. E., Bond, R. N., Cohen, J., & Stein, M. (1989). Major depressive disorder and immunity: Role of age, sex, severity and hospitalization. *Archives of General Psychiatry, 46,* 81–87.

Scrambler, G., & Hopkins, A. (1986). Being epileptic, coming to terms with stigma. *Sociology of Health and Illness, 8,* 26–43.

Segerstrom, S. C., & Miller, A. (2004). Psychological stress and the human immune system: A meta-analytic study of 30 years of inquiry. *Psychological Bulletin, 130,* 601–630.

Selye, K. (1976). *The stress of life.* New York: McGraw-Hill.

Sen, A. (2000). *Social exclusion: Concept, application, and scrutiny.* Social Development Bank Paper 1, Asian Development Bank.

Shah, V. P., Seth, N. R., & Visaria, P. (1998). Swadhyaya: Social change through spirituality. In M. L. Dantawala, H. Sethi & P. Visaria (Eds.), *Social change through voluntary action* (pp. 57–73). New Delhi: SAGE Publications.

Shankar, D. (1992). Indigenous health services: The state of the art. In A. Mukhopadhyay (Ed.), *State of India's health.* New Delhi: Voluntary Health Association of India.

Sharma, S. (1981). Key concepts of social psychology in India. *Psychologia, 24,* 105–114.

———. (1999). Social support, stress and psychological well-being. In G. Misra (Ed.), *Psychological perspectives on stress and health* (pp. 126–146). New Delhi: Concept.

———. (2007). Community participation in community-based rehabilitation programmes. *Asia Pacific Disability Rehabilitation Journal, 18*(2), 146–157.

Sharma, S., & Misra, G. (2009). Health psychology: Progress and challenges. In G. Misra (Ed.), *Psychology in India* (Vol. 4). New Delhi: Pearson.

Shiraev, E. (2010). *A history of psychology: A global perspective.* London: SAGE Publications.

Sri Aurobindo. (1997). *Collected works of Sri Aurobindo* (Vol. 22). Puducherry: Aurobindo Ashram.

Shweder, R. (1991). *Thinking through cultures: Expeditions in cultural psychology.* Cambridge: Harvard University Press.

Siegel, B. S. (1986). *Love, medicine and miracles.* London: Arrow Books.

Simpson, L. (2001). Aboriginal people and knowledge: Decolonizing our processes. *The Canadian Journal of Native Studies, 21,* 37–48.

Sinha, D. (1990). Concept of psychological well-being: Western and Indian perspectives. *NIMHANS Journal, 8,* 1–11.

Smith, J. A. (2004). *Qualitative psychology: A practical guide to research methods.* London. SAGE Publications.

Smith, L. T. (2012). *Decolonizing methodologies: Research and indigenous peoples* (2nd Edition). London and New York: Zed Books.

Snyder, C., & Lopez, S. (1999). *Handbook of positive psychology.* New York: Oxford University Press.

Snyder, C. R., & Lopez, S. J. (Eds.) (2002). *The handbook of positive psychology.* New York: Oxford University Press.

Solberg Nes, L., & Segerstrom, S. C. (2006). Dispositional optimism and coping: A meta-analytic review. *Personality and Social Psychology Review, 10,* 235–251.

Srivastava, A. K., & Misra, G. (2011). Happiness and well-being: An Indian perspective. In G. Misra (Ed.), *Handbook of psychology in India* (pp. 299–310). New Delhi: Oxford University Press.

Stafford, M. C., & Scott, R. R. (1986). Stigma deviance and social control: Some conceptual issues. In S. C. Ainlay, G. Becker & L. M. Coleman (Eds.), *The dilemma of difference.* New York: Plenum.

Stoppard, J. M. (2002). Navigating the hazards of orthodox: Introducing a graduate course on qualitative methods into psychology curriculum. *Canadian Psychology, 43,* 143–153.

Stretcher, V. J., & Rosenstock, I. M. (1997). The health belief model. In A. Baum (Ed.), *Cambridge handbook of psychology, health and medicine* (pp. 113–117). Cambridge, UK: Cambridge University Press.

Svoboda, R. E. (1992). *Ayurveda: Life, health and longevity.* New Delhi: Penguin Books.

Swami Satchidanand (2008). *The yoga sutra of Patanjali.* Yogville, VA: Satchidanand Ashram.

Tankha, A. (2002). *Self-help groups as financial intermediaries in India: Cost of promotion, sustainability and impact.* A study prepared for ICCO and Cordaid, The Netherlands.

Taylor, S. E. (1983). Adjustment to threatening events. *American Psychologist, 38,* 1161–1173.

———. (1989). *Positive illusions: Creative self-deception and the healthy mind.* New York: Basic Books.

———. (2006). *Health psychology.* New Delhi: Tata Mcgraw Hill.

Thomas, P. (2005a). *Disability, poverty and the millennium development goals: Relevance, challenges and opportunities for DFID.* London: DFID Disability KaR Programme.

———. (2005b). *Poverty reduction and development in Cambodia: Enabling disabled to play a role.* Disability KaR, April 2005. Retrieved from http://www.disabilitykar. net/pdfs/cambodia.pdf on 8 August 2013.

Thomas, R. M. (2001). *Folk psychologies across cultures.* New Delhi: SAGE Publications.

Tripathi, R. C., & Sinha, Y. (Eds.). (2013). *Psychology as a policy science.* New Delhi: Springer.

Tudawe, I. (2001). *Chronic poverty and development policy in Sri Lanka.* Chronic Poverty Research Centre Working Paper 9. Institute of Development Policy and Management/CPRC, Manchester.

Uchino, B. N., Uno, D., & Holt-Lunstad, J. (1999). Social support, physiological processes, and health. *Current Directions in Psychological Science, 8,* 145–148.

UNAIDS. (2001). *Comparative Analysis: Research studies from India and Uganda: HIV and AIDS-related Stigma, Discrimination and Denial.* UNAIDS, Geneva. Retrieved from http://www.unaids.org/publications/documents/human/law/ugandaindi-aBB.pdf on 8 August 2013.

UNESCO (United Nations Educational, Scientific and Cultural Organization. (2005). *Education for all: Monitoring report.* UNESCO, Paris.

Vaillant, G. E., & Mukamal, K. (2001). Successful aging. *American Journal of Psychiatry, 158,* 839–847.

Valsiner, J. (2007). *Culture in minds and societies: Foundation of cultural psychology.* New Delhi: SAGE Publications.

Vanderpool, H. Y. (1977). Is religion therapeutically significant? *Journal of Religious Health, 16,* 255–259.

Varela, F., & Shear, J. (Eds.). (1999). *The view from within: First person approaches to the study of consciousness.* UK: Imprint Academic.

Verma, S. K., & Verma, A. (1989). *Manual for PGI general wellbeing measure.* Lucknow: Ankur Psychological Agency. VHAI. (1991). *India's health status.* New Delhi: Voluntary Health Association of India.

Visvanathan, S. (1997). *A carnival for survival: Essays on science, technology and development.* New Delhi: Oxford University Press.

Vyas, T. J. (1998). Community living in rural Andhra: A study of social cohesiveness. *Journal of Community Living, 3,* 61–70.

Wade, D. T. (2004). Do biomedical model of illness make good care system? *British Medical Journal, 329*(7479), 1398–1401.

Watts, A. (1975). *Psychotherapy east and west.* New York: Vintage Books.

Weiss, G. L., & Lonnquist, L. E. (1996). *The sociology of health, healing and illness.* New Jersey: Prentice Hall.

Werner, D. (2009). *Disabled village children.* Berkeley, CA: Hesperian Society.

Wetzel, M. S., Eisenberg, D. M., & Kaptchuk, T. J. (September 1998). Courses involving complementary and alternative medicine at US medical schools. *Journal of American Medical Association, 280* (9), 784–787.

Williams, C. (2003). Vulnerable victims? A current awareness of the victimisation of people with learning disabilities. *Disability, Handicap and Society, 8*(2), 161–172.

World Bank Disability Policy Center. (2005). *Disability and Development and the World Bank—A Briefing Summary on February 2, 2005.* Washington, D.C.: World Bank.

World Bank Report. (2008, December 3). *People with disability in India: From commitments to outcomes.* Washington, D.C.: World Bank.

World Health Organization (WHO). (1978). *Alma–Ata declaration.* Geneva: WHO.

———. (1980). *International classification of impairments, disabilities, and handicaps.* Geneva: WHO.

———. (1998). *Annual report.* Geneva: WHO.

———. (2001). *International classification of functioning, disability and health: introduction.* Geneva: WHO.

———. (2005). *Annual report 2005.* Geneva: WHO.

———. (2011). *Annual report.* Geneva: WHO.

Wortman, C. B. (1983). Coping with victimization: Conclusions and implications for future research. *Journal of Social Issues, 39*(2), 195–221.

Wright, B. A. (1983). *Physical disability: A psychological approach.* New York: Harper and Row.

Yeo, R. (2005). *Disability, poverty, and the new development agenda: Disability Knowledge and Research Programme.* Retrieved from http://www.dfid.gov.uk/r4d/PDF/Outputs/Disa on 8 August 2013.

Yeo, R., & Moore, K. (2003). Including disabled people in poverty reduction work: Nothing about us, without us. *World Development, 31*(3), 571–590.

Zimmer, H. (1951).*Philosophies of India.* Princeton, NJ: Princeton University.

Zimmerman, F. (1999). *The jungle and the aroma of meats, an ecological theme in Hindu medicine.* Varanasi: Motilal Banarasidas.

Zysk, K. G. (1998). *Asceticism and healing in India: Medicine in the Buddhist monastery.* New Delhi: Motilal Banarasidass.

Index

About the Author

Ajit K Dalal is currently Writer-in Residence at the Mahatma Gandhi Antarrashtriya Hindi Vishwavidyalaya, Wardha, Maharashtra. He has recently retired as a professor of psychology from the University of Allahabad. He was the Head of Psychology Department (2011–2012) and had held several other academic positions at the university. He was the editor of an international journal, *Psychology and Developing Societies* (2001–2011). He is also on editorial boards of several other journals.

Professor Dalal received the Fulbright Senior Fellowship in 1982. He worked at the University of California, Los Angeles and at the University of Michigan, Ann Arbor. He is also a recipient of the University Grants Commission's (UGC) Career Award (1990–1993), Rockefeller Foundation Award (1992) and the Senior Research Fellowship (1998 and 2012) from Indian Council of Social Science Research (ICSSR). He was an adjunct professor at Queen's University, Canada (1992–1998) and was a visiting faculty at several institutions, including National Institute of Health and Family Welfare, New Delhi; Indian Institute of Management, Ahmedabad and University of Calcutta, Kolkata.

Professor Dalal has published his work in the areas such as causal attribution, health beliefs and healing traditions of India and Indian psychology. He has published about 95 research articles and book chapters. He has also published several books; prominent among them are: *Attribution Theory and Research* (1988), *New Directions in Indian Psychology* (Vol. 1) (with G. Misra, 2002), *Social Dimensions of Health* (with S. Ray, 2005), *Handbook of Indian Psychology* (with K. R. Rao and A. C. Paranjpe, 2008), *New Directions in Health Psychology* (with G. Misra, 2011), *Qualitative Research on Well-Being and Self-Growth: Contemporary Indian Perspectives* (with R. Priya, 2014) and *Health Beliefs and Coping with Chronic Diseases* (2015).